Good Girls D

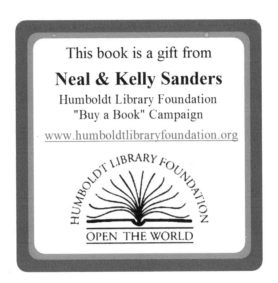
A memoir by

Patti Hawn

In *Good Girls Don't*, Patti Hawn brings aliveness, excitement and a mystical quality into a life fully lived. Coming from a family that has given birth to many creatives, she finds her voice in the written word with insights into self, family, loss, forgiveness and ultimately redemption.

> **Ronald A. Alexander, Ph.D.**, Author of *Wise Mind, Open Mind,* Director of Open Mind Training Institute, Santa Monica, CA.

Patti Hawn's story takes us to a place of innocent intimacy. She captures a life-altering event in a beautifully told balance of descriptive detail and uncanny purity of emotion. She accomplishes this — not just in the retelling — but in "original" time. Her style is simple and yet, elegantly honest and true. This is an important story: It lays bare the profound and often primal connections we all carry deeply within us. Patti's story inspires us to know that we can always go back, can always complete that which we had thought unfinished and lost to us for good. The past can be rewritten, and more importantly, reclaimed.

> **Abigail Brenner, MD**, Psychiatrist, Author of *Transitions: How Women Embrace Change and Celebrate Life* and *SHIFT: How to Deal When Life Changes.*

Totally evocative of an era that is an example of why some "traditions" (often concerning women) are best left in the dust. The story is very moving - revealing one astounding event after another. It peels back the pages of what must have been an incredibly painful time in an innocent girl's life. If you think you know what this book is about, you are probably wrong.

> **Deana Newcomb**, Motion Picture Photographer whose credits include *Twilight, Waiting for Guffman, The Alamo.*

What a ride! This is a book that makes you think and feel and no reader will remain untouched by this real life journey. I was hooked from the first page by the vivid descriptions and total honesty that Patti so generously and openly shares with us about her life, choices, and family secrets. From beginning to end this book is nothing short of AMAZING!

> **Rita Battat Silverman,** Talent manager

Good Girls Don't

Dear Son,

    I said good-bye to you many years ago. You were small and helpless and so was I. It didn't seem like a very good match, so I did what seemed like a good idea at the time: I gave you away. I thought you would have a better chance in this life with two parents who were married, who had a home and could afford to give you the so-called "advantages" that were so revered in the fifties. There was a lot of support for this at the time. My mother, your grandmother was a take-charge kind of lady who when presented with a problem, took action. In this case, the action was adoption. I was told it would be an incredibly selfish act on my part to consider anything else. By the time the decision was made I was actually feeling rather noble about my gift — of you.

    I dropped out of school, created a past that included a husband, moved to Pittsburgh for seven months with a kind family member and watched in awe as you grew inside my body. You and I spent many hours in the library visiting exotic places and reading stories of people who became my friends and teachers. I don't expect you remember, but I always hoped you would love to read and learn. I used to massage your tiny knees and elbows as they rippled across my belly while you tried to find your spot inside of me. I watched in fascination as you changed my young girl's body into that of a woman. My breasts grew large and full in preparation for the milk you never drank. I shared many secrets with you in those months.

I told you I would always be with you, although you might not know it, and each year on October 18th I would have a birthday party for you. I told you about your unique and talented family — starting with your Southern grandfather, who played music for kings and presidents, who could make a violin weep and a clarinet laugh, and your tiny Jewish grandmother, a master storyteller whose smile was so radiant and eyes so wise she enchanted all who touched her life. I told you of your beautiful young aunt who could hold an arabesque longer than anyone in our dancing class, who was just beginning an extraordinary journey that would lead her throughout the world and into the hearts of millions. I told you of the young boy who was your father. He had a kind laugh and a keen mind. I knew he would grow up to be a scholar. And he did.

As for me: my favorite color is yellow. I'll eat almost anything except raw oysters; I've always owned a dog and wouldn't live in a house without a fireplace. I love the sea but need to feel trees often. I don't much like boats, Brazilian jazz makes my body move and I can't imagine anything more thrilling than getting on a plane to visit somewhere I've never been. I have a husband who makes me laugh almost all the time and two sons who constantly teach me about love. There isn't too much that scares me except maybe the thought of never seeing you. I made a promise long ago to remain silent in your life, and I have, for 40 years. Now I break my silence and my promise. I want nothing from you but to look into your eyes, touch your face and know that you are safe.

Love,
Patti.

Good Girls Don't

PART I

Lost

CHAPTER 1

In my sharpest memory I am surrounded by dark. I sit at the top of the stairs and listen. Sounds are harsh. Angry voices rise and fall. I am compelled to stay, huddled into the corner of the hallway night after night, commanding my post like a small sentry. Wrapped in a blanket, I huddle against the banister, straining to hear every word. I tuck my bare feet under my white flannel nightgown dotted with yellow daisies, and strain to hear. Her voice, loud and commanding. His, softer, yielding, often slurred. My breathing feels shallow. They must not hear me. If I am discovered I may be devoured. I store their rage in my tiny body and hide it away in a secret place to be protected at all cost. If my hiding place is revealed, I will surely vanish and never be seen again.

DADDY WAS A MUSICIAN WHO EARNED his living playing the violin, clarinet and saxophone. Most nights after dinner, when the parents of my friends were preparing to spend an evening listening to Jack Benny or Fred Allen on the radio, my father was putting on a tuxedo and going to work. It's funny, I never remember hearing him play much at home. I guess he figured he performed enough outside. Daddy used to hang his tuxedo pants by his suspenders on the edge of his closet door and lie down for a quick nap before going to work. I can still see the long black pants dancing on the edge of the door, like the tall man on stilts leading the circus parade. "Be still, Daddy's lying down," Mom would say. And I knew the radio had to be turned down and he could not be disturbed. Daddy's catnaps were admirable. He could fall asleep in thirty seconds and be snoring in a minute flat.

The smell of garlic often woke me at midnight. It never seemed particularly odd to me that Daddy would be cooking garlic in the middle of the night. He went on food jags, cooking and eating one particular dish for months at a time and then, suddenly, garlic and oil over spaghetti would end, Tex-Mex would begin and chili peppers would replace garlic as my midnight wake-up call.

The drama of my family always played out in the middle of the night. I would hear the refrigerator open and ice hit the glass, and I would settle into my corner in the hallway for the theater of my family to begin. The theme of their bickering was commonplace, even banal. He drank too much. There wasn't enough money. He was too weak. She didn't want to be strong. It was not the subject that was notable but rather the flair and color with which they fought. Their arguments were like drive-by shootings. They seemed to draw delight in taking each other to the edge of control with gilded bullets that rarely missed their mark.

If they were the stars, I was their audience. Sometimes, before being banished to bed, I would sit in the back room, as we called it, enveloped in a large brown overstuffed corduroy chair: the same chair where Spotty, my Dalmatian and confidante, delivered her litter. They seemed oblivious to my presence. Perhaps they played better to an audience, even if it was a seven-year old. I burrowed deep into the folds of the soft chair and allowed the corduroy to swaddle me as I sensed that their performance was about to begin. Even at the age of seven, I did not want to miss a moment of the pageant. I knew my role and played it well.

We were the first family in our neighborhood to get a television set. Daddy, who was an artist and probably had never paid attention to a wrestling match in his life, became fascinated with television wrestling. He and I watched together as Gorgeous George and The Flying Dutchman pummeled each other with outrageous drama. One night when I was about eight or nine, he came home from work early to prepare for a grand night of wrestling. After I was grown I was amazed to recall how detached I'd been as a child from my father's strange rituals. He carefully placed his tuxedo jacket on the back of the dining room chair and went to the kitchen, where he took the scotch bottle from the top shelf in the cupboard and poured some into a water glass. He then opened the refrigerator and selected an array of bottles and jars of condiments including Worcester sauce, Tabasco, horseradish, and—when we had it—a jar of small stuffed olives, the kind dotted with tiny red pimentos. He unfolded the black metal TV tray and carefully placed it beside the rocking chair in our back room. Then he brought in the drinks and open jars and arranged them on the tray. He kicked off his shiny black shoes and, oblivious to the scent of his freshly unbound feet, settled in for a night of pleasure. He studied the condiments, selected one and put it to his nose, taking in the aroma. His pinky finger, delicately pointed upward, would rise to the occasion directly in proportion to the amount of scotch he consumed. Immediately after allowing himself this sensual pleasure he would take a large swallow of scotch, and the games began. It never occurred to me that this was remotely unusual, and to my recollection nobody ever asked him why he did it. I guess I thought everybody's father sniffed horseradish.

I can't remember exactly what my mother was angry about. I guess her life didn't turn out the way she had dreamed it would. This was often the theme of her discontent, and she spoke on the subject eloquently. During one of the sip-and-smell evenings, Daddy, a master of avoidance, could take no more of her ranting.

He rose elegantly from the rocking chair and without emotion fetched the Electrolux vacuum cleaner. He plugged it in and, holding his finger over the switch like a brilliant commander at war, drowned her out with the roar. Each time she began speaking, he would flick the switch with Fred Astaire nonchalance. Mom's mouth tightened into a hard line in an attempt to swallow the giggle that could not be stopped, and finally, when her laughter escaped into our back room, my heart soared and I knew I was safe — at least for a while. She could never defend herself from his most skillful weapon, his humor.

My father, a talented musician, celebrated as a child prodigy, really aspired to only one thing: he desperately wanted to be a member of the Kiwanis Club. I think he felt this honor would give him the respectability that his artistry never could. Born in El Dorado, Arkansas, in 1910 to Claire Estelle Johnson, a piano teacher, and O.D. Hawn, a teletyper for the railroad, he showed early talent as a violinist. He received scholarships to some of the finest music conservatories of the time and attended the Cincinnati Conservatory of Music when he was 16. His name was Edward Rutledge Hawn, after the youngest signer of the Declaration of Independence, but I never heard him called anything but "Rut." My sister and I shared many laughs over our proper southern lineage, which allowed us membership in the "Daughters of The American Revolution," the same organization that banned Marian Anderson from performing at Constitution Hall in 1939 in Washington, D.C. because she was an African American.

By the time Daddy reached Washington, D.C., in 1934, he had left school, joined a traveling band and played in backroom saloons in Texas, speakeasies in Chicago and one-night stands in Oklahoma. When he arrived in New York City he became the music director for Arthur Godfrey and sat in with Tommy Dorsey and many of the Big Band leaders of the day. There were rumors

Good Girls Don't

of a love affair with a statuesque blonde showgirl named Sonny Dale, who Mom allegedly met years later. Mom loved to tell the story of placing me in Sonny's arms at three months old and gloating as I threw up on the poor woman's sequined dress.

My parents met at Shannon's Boarding House in Washington, D.C., in 1935. He was playing at the Hi-Ho Club, a hip nightclub frequented by sparkling names of the entertainment, diplomatic and political worlds. My mother, a dark, curvaceous small-town beauty, had been raised in an Orthodox Jewish family outside of Pittsburgh. She escaped the depression by moving to Washington, D.C., and finding a job with the Interior Department as a clerk. My father — a southern, introverted, aristocratic WASP — and my tiny, vivacious mother tested every aspect of the institution of marriage. Although she was something of a rebel, she never really strayed too far from her traditions. She lied to her family, telling them Daddy was Jewish, and reminding them that they needed to be patient with him because Southern Jews were different.

In the second grade I fell in love with my father. It was an autumn morning — the kind of golden morning I've unsuccessfully searched for in many places since leaving Maryland years ago. Orange and gold leaves chased each other in our front yard and the crisp air held the promise of magic around every corner.

In my haste to be on time for school, I forgot my new baseball jacket. It was a green and white satin warm-up jacket that I had begged my parents to buy me for months, and I had chosen it to take that morning for "show and tell." The show-and-tell portion of our day began early, and I sadly took my seat in the back of the classroom with nothing to offer. I was concentrating on Miss Freeman's plaid, pleated skirt, bravely trying to keep back my tears, when Daddy burst through the classroom door with the jacket flung over his arm. He was wearing a blue sweater, the color of sky, that matched his eyes. He was on his way to play an early job somewhere downtown. He marched right through Miss Freeman's class to the back where I was seated and put the jacket around my shoulders. Judy Levine, who was in the front of the class, clutching her gold fish bowl, and who, only moments before, had loudly suggested that I really didn't have a warm-up jacket, but had made it all up, stopped talking and stared at Daddy. Everyone stared at him. It was the first time I realized how handsome he was. He gave me a secret wink, smiled at Miss Freeman, who smiled back broadly in a grown-up, knowing kind of way, and was gone. I remember Miss Freeman asking me after class if that was my father. She said he looked too young to be anybody's father. He was shiny and golden that day, not unlike the autumn morning. Another reason, perhaps, why I've always loved autumn best of all seasons.

Good Girls Don't

CHAPTER 2

I sit on the edge of the tub, watching you put on your make-up, a ritual I never tire of witnessing. Your lipstick is always bright red. The tube touches your lips boldly, first outlining your upper lip and then carefully tracing the full line of your lower lip. Your dark eyes gaze into the small bathroom mirror with the fixed stare of a surgeon. My mouth moves automatically with yours; in that moment my transference to you is complete. You smile and your perfect white teeth glisten. It is here that my comparison to you begins. I am thin and angular with straight, red hair. You are small, curvy, with curly dark hair. You are the ideal. I am the counterfeit. I linger in the bathroom and take your place at the mirror. I secretly try to imitate your seductive smile and your hooded dark eyes. All I see is a pale, thin little girl, and wonder: where have I really come from?

MY MOTHER, A LARGE WOMAN trapped inside a small body, filled up rooms without ever saying a word. I can still hear the sound her tiny feet made when she hit the floor to begin her day. I usually heard it in the twilight before sleep took me into dreams, or when I first awakened and the day stretched ahead, unformed. Mom's sound was always urgent, immediate. Even now, whenever I sense her moving through a room, I feel as though whatever

I'm doing, I should be doing something else — something more, better or just different. Fabergé perfume clung to her body and our home. There was never any mistaking her presence.

If I learned the unexpected from my father, Mom taught me order. I learned how to hang sheets up on a clothesline so taut they never needed to be ironed and smelled like fresh spring air. I learned how to make a bed with neat corners tucked underneath the mattress so it always felt smooth and newly made. I learned to put icicles on a Christmas tree one at a time and not throw them carelessly so they hung in messy clumps, and to name all the spring wildflowers that grew in our backyard. Mom taught me how to crunch newspapers into tight balls and place them under kindling wood to light roaring fires in our large stone fireplace. And it was from Mom that I learned to listen. She was a storyteller. There was a time when her stories became mine and I wasn't sure where hers ended and mine began.

Her stage was our knotty-pine back room and her props were a coffee cup filled with instant Nescafé and a pack of Camel cigarettes. Fragments of her rush in upon me as I recall her tales:

"Tanta Goldie took me in when I was only three years old. My father didn't know what to do with a little girl after my mother died, so he dropped me off at Tanta Goldie's and Uncle Joe's and I lived with them in a house in Uniontown outside of Pittsburgh. Kids used to tease me because I only spoke Yiddish. Tanta Goldie never let me call her "Ma" like the rest of the kids, but I know she loved me anyway. My father would visit me a couple of times a year, and I still remember how excited I got when I saw him coming down the street. He brought me beautiful clothes. I never knew where he found such fine clothes, but I was always the best-dressed little girl in town. He made sure of that. Your grandfather's name was Max. The rest of the family never liked him much. Tanta Sarah said he hit my mother and that's why she died. I never believed it. She died in childbirth. "They used to tell me he drank but I never saw it. His watch repair shop was the place where all the men in town would congregate and tell stories about the old country. Did you know your grandfather could speak four languages?"

This was usually the part when she sat back in her chair and took a long thoughtful drag on her cigarette, and I knew she was lost somewhere deep inside of a past—one where, although I was invited, I could never really visit. The audience that I provided her was no longer necessary. She needed to tell her stories like most people need air. The tales of her life were filled with images of Zayde drinking coffee from a jelly glass in the kitchen and Tanta Goldie sitting at the window of the big walk-up apartment where they lived in Braddock, where Mom had been raised by Tanta Goldie.

"Tanta Goldie was pregnant with Allen, her seventh child, when she saw Anne Petranak's boyfriend stab a man in the street, right outside her window. She clutched her belly so hard it left a birthmark shaped like a strawberry on the baby's back."

Family was always central to her theme. It wasn't until many years later that it struck me as odd that she'd married a man so removed from everything familiar to her.

"I thought your father was a waiter when I first met him at the boarding house," she used to like to say. "He always had on a tuxedo and never was around in the morning—so what should I think?

It was the radio that first woke me this Saturday night. The radio was in my parents' bedroom at the end of the hall—the hall where the monsters lived inside the walls during the day, but came out at night and played tricks on anyone not in their beds with the covers tightly pulled up. I can't remember exactly when Daddy began keeping the radio on all night, but I think it began about the same time his legs started to hurt.

"Rut, you're sick," Mom pleaded. "You need a specialist. Maybe there's a test that'll find where the pain comes from. You look awful. Do something, anything. You can't go on like this." She burst into sobs and ran downstairs to the back room.

He said nothing, but turned up the volume. It doesn't matter what station was playing or who was singing or talking. He never allowed it to be turned off. He got up to go to the bathroom, and that was when I first saw the red welts on his legs. I remembered thinking that the welts must have come from the demons who lived inside the walls in our upstairs hallway. Then I realized that the purple bruises came from him pinching himself in attempts to stop the pain.

Daddy eventually went to doctors and had many tests, but no answers. As quickly as a test would dispel any possibility of a physical problem in his legs the pain would move to his arms, or head, or hands. Pretty soon there were no more spots left to hurt. Daddy went to Florida. It was the first time I heard the word "psychosomatic."

Daddy opened the watch-repair shop soon after our flight into the suburbs. He moved the tall bench that held my grandfather's tools out of the basement into the store in Takoma Park and set up business. Daddy's view of the world was confined to the inside of a watch that he studied with Zen-like concentration. He put on his black eyepiece and shut out everything beyond the intricate works of a timepiece. Maybe he found answers in this tiny world, answers that escaped him when he performed on stage.

It was Mom, however, who ran the business. She bought Elgin watches, gold-link watchbands and strands of pearls to put inside the store window. The shop became a place for people to have their watches cleaned and gossip about religion and politics. My mother had opinions on everything and shared them at a moment's notice. She charmed her way into the Chamber of Commerce and soon became the vice-president. Daddy played fewer music jobs, and soon moved into a second shop when the store proved too small for the two of them. He escaped into its tiny confines where Mom supplied him enough watches to fix to keep us going. The tuxedo stopped dancing on his closet door, replaced with a sport jacket and tie. And Daddy became a member of the Silver Spring Kiwanis Club.

Daddy arrived home for dinner one night after returning from the shop. Mom was the kitchen pounding flour into a piece of round steak with the edge of a plate. Her eyes were red from onions she'd sliced and put into the frying pan. I was carefully folding paper napkins into triangles to be placed under the silverware. (Regardless of what we were eating for dinner, a small salad plate always sat to the right of the knife, filled with a spoonful of cottage cheese inside a canned peach half, topped by a maraschino cherry.) Daddy went directly upstairs to lie down for a nap before dinner when Mom told me to wake him.

"Tell your mother I'm not hungry and need to rest," he mumbled.

"But we're having Swiss steak for dinner," I said.

Daddy turned on the radio, closed his eyes and pulled the covers up under his chin.

Dr. Cohen arrived at our house later that night, carried his black bag into the bedroom and closed the door. Daddy stayed in bed for a long time after that.

I was ten years old when I hid the scotch bottle in the basement. Daddy had left for work and Mom and I settled into our cozy back room in front of a blazing fire, where the turquoise walls had been exchanged for knotty pine paneling, to watch Milton Berle on television, as we did every Tuesday night.

Mom tucked her feet underneath her and settled into the corner of the couch. She took an exaggerated drag on her cigarette and blew it out in a long stream and I nestled into the big corduroy chair near the television set.

"Sometimes I feel like these walls are closing in on me," Mom began, staring off into the smoke that swirled above her head. She didn't really look at me while she talked, but I knew I was expected to listen.

"I just want to pick you up and run somewhere. It used to be so different. I used to be something before I met your father. Did you know I was the one in my crowd who was the most fun-loving? I could stay up dancing all night and be fresh as a daisy for work the next morning. When I first came to Washington, Henry Caton, a circuit court judge, asked me to marry him. His brother, Harry, was a dentist who kept my picture in his office and told everyone he'd made my teeth because they were so perfect."

Meanwhile, on television, Milton Berle wore a dress and danced with Lucille Ball. Everybody in the audience was laughing. I kept looking at Mom. Every time she took a sip from her coffee cup, I stole a peek at Uncle Miltie. I wanted Mom to stop talking so I could hear the jokes.

"Your father really doesn't know what it's like to be part of a family," she continued. "I don't think he's really an alcoholic, because he can't hold his liquor. He gets sick right away. I think alcoholics can actually drink more than he does. It jiggles something in his brain, though, that's for sure. Believe it or not, your father is a prude. The only time he lets his hair down is when he's drinking. I told him the other day I was going to take you and move out. Of course he wouldn't know what to do without us. He seems to get worse every time his mother calls. I don't know what went on with that family, but it's stuff I'll never understand. You know, I'm the one who has to get up early and open the store while he's up frying garlic until two in the morning. I wake up to a kitchen disaster before my eyes are even open. You know the truth is he'd probably be better off by himself. He's a very introverted man and I'm extremely extroverted. So there you have it."

By this time Mom was off on her own reverie and deep into a one-way conversation. "That's it in a nutshell. I hope you learn something from all this. Sometimes I think that Florida was the happiest time of my life," she continued. " I should have stayed there. I've never felt so free and young. All your father does is hand me a comb whenever we go anywhere. Do you know how that feels when someone does that to you? Oh, what's the use, things won't change. Remember what I tell you." At this point her voice dropped to almost a whisper: "Things never get any better, they just get a little worse. You start off with the first fight and you can never take it back, and the next time you say something a little worse, and on and on and on."

"Honey," Mom said, looking at me as though she'd just discovered I was in the room. "Put some more water on to boil for coffee and bring in the batch of fudge from the fridge."

My heart sank when Mom got up from the couch to turn the volume down on the television set. All I saw was Milton Berle, in drag, dancing with a line of chorus girls and the audience going mad, applauding. I walked into the kitchen to get the candy she'd made earlier for our Tuesday night with Uncle Miltie.

The next morning before I left for school, I climbed up on the kitchen counter and pulled down the bottle of scotch. I hid it in the basement on a dusty shelf, behind the laundry basket filled with the clean sheets. Mom and Daddy were still asleep so the house was very still. I returned to my cocoa and cinnamon toast and picked up the comics in the morning paper to see what Orphan Annie was up to. Maybe now Mom would watch Milton Berle with me.

The following week, after I'd gone to bed, Daddy came into my bedroom and sat on the edge of my bed. His face looked tired and his voice was quiet.

"Did you take the bottle of liquor into the basement?" he asked.

I looked out my bedroom window into the darkness and tried to breathe, but couldn't seem to find air. I couldn't look into his eyes, they hurt too much. I wished more than anything I'd taken the bottle out of the basement and put it back on the top shelf where it belonged. I guess I knew hiding the bottle wouldn't make Mom feel pretty again or make Daddy stop being an introvert, which I figured must be a pretty bad thing to be. I just wanted them to stop fighting with each other.

One day, years later, Daddy just stopped drinking. There were no family interventions with people writing him heartfelt letters about his indiscretions. No mention of Alcoholics Anonymous or even a declaration of sobriety on his part. It was apparently a quiet, private decision that, to my knowledge, he never discussed with anyone.

He stopped playing music for five years, devoting his time to the watch-repair business. After he returned from his rest in Florida, Mom made a clandestine phone call to his music agent, urging him to seduce Daddy back into the business of being a musician. His violin and saxophone cases once again were propped up in the hallway by the front door and Daddy never knew that Mom had made that call.

"Rut, man, we need you," said Sidney, Daddy's agent. "Let Laura run the shop for awhile and come back and play a few jobs. It'll be good for you. The guys down at the White House keep asking for you. They say Jack Kennedy's going to win this election and you know how those guys like to party. We'll all get rich off of that action."

Daddy relented and soon the tuxedo was dancing again. The pains that had driven him to doctors and medical tests and eventually to rest in Florida vanished. Mom became the vice-president of the Takoma Park Chamber of Commerce and Daddy returned to his music.

It's funny how sometimes photographs become memories, and you can't remember whether you recall the event or the photo. I have one of these shots of Mom wearing a dirndl skirt and peasant blouse, posing in front of a cottage in St. Petersburg, Florida. One hand rested on her hip and the other pointed inside an empty mailbox. She looked like a pin-up girl in an old war poster. It was 1944 and Mom had left Daddy after a particularly bad fight about his drinking. She had a new friend, a dancer named Roberta, also married to a musician. Roberta had lived in New York and danced on Broadway. She was glamorous and sophisticated and taught Mom how to pile her hair on top of her head in an upsweep like Rita Hayworth. After the fight it was Roberta who urged Mom to pack up our things and go down to Florida for a rest, to "think things through." She had a friend from New York who owned a cottage we could use as long as we wanted, so two months before my fourth birthday the three of us boarded a train for Florida. St. Petersburg had not yet become a playground for the old, but was filled with khaki uniforms, bomber planes and young women with bright red lipstick. It bustled with men and women living their lives as though they had very little time – and sadly, this was all too often true. Mom flourished there. I have a memory — or maybe it's a dream, it doesn't matter — of her standing before a mirror, swaying to the rhythm of a popular song played on every radio station during that time called *Tangerine*. She moved her hips to the sounds of the moist, sultry voice, threw her head back and sang with the radio. It was my birthday and Mom promised me a cake with candles — but first, she danced over to the refrigerator, her black hair falling to her shoulders, her tiny compact body the color of terra cotta, and swooped me into her arms. I giggled and snuggled into her scent of orange blossoms as we danced through the tiny cottage. Sounds of planes overhead buzzed our bungalow like huge protective hawks. Mom threw open the screen door and waved to the Florida sky. Her voice sounded deep and throaty; I waved too, and the B-17 bomber tilted its wings, saluting our cottage. My fourth birthday was the color of tangerines.

CHAPTER 3

I WAS SEVEN YEARS OLD WHEN MY SISTER WAS BORN.
Family folklore suggested I willed her into the world through my
heartfelt bedtime prayers. "…and please bring me a little brother
or sister…" I would whisper, with solemn reverence. "I don't care
what kind," I begged, "I'm the only kid in school without one. It's
embarrassing."

There was never any question surrounding the unusual
choice of Goldie's name. It was chosen in honor of the aunt who
raised Mom and died several months prior to my sister's arrival.
My mother, who was among the most pragmatic women I've ever
known, reluctantly confided to us years later that Tanta Goldie had
come to her in a dream while she was pregnant and told her that
her daughter would make the name Goldie famous.

People have asked me throughout the years what it's like to
have a famous sister and I usually offer the glib reply, "I don't
know what it's like not to have one." But, in fact, this is a lie. I distinctly remembered the feeling of holding center stage during
those first seven years of my life — before she was born.

At the same time Truman dropped the bomb ending the
Second World War, Goldie was rehearsing her entrance into the

world. I was unprepared for the explosion her arrival would create in my young life. I was both fascinated and annoyed by her intrusion into my domain. What seemed like a good idea during bedtime prayers proved to turn my life upside-down.

It was a cold November morning in 1945 when Daddy drove into the driveway with Mom holding a bundled-up tiny baby in her arms. I had spent the morning taking up a collection of pennies from the neighborhood kids to welcome my new baby sister with a gift. I waited on the front porch with the 87 cents I'd collected, wrapped in pink tissue paper, when they pulled up in Daddy's big blue Lincoln. Mom's young cousin, Ruth, one of Aunt Goldie's eight children, had arrived the day before from Pittsburgh to help out while Mom got back on her feet. I followed them up the stairs into my parents' bedroom, where Daddy placed Goldie inside a wicker bassinet and Mom crawled into bed. Mom placed the gift on the dresser and assured me she loved it, but all the attention was focused on the baby. I sat on the bed and watched Ruth, Mom and Daddy stand over the bassinet studying the sleeping Goldie as though she was doing something remarkable. I do that every night, I thought. Looking back, I wonder if I sensed — even then — that watching my sister being watched was something I'd do a lot.

I'd missed Mom while she was in the hospital. I wanted to tell her about the spelling bee I'd almost won at school and the new girl in my class who'd become my friend, but she needed sleep because, I guessed, getting a baby made her really tired.

"Go play in your room," said Ruth, taking charge. "Your mom needs to rest while the baby's sleeping."

"You're not my boss," I mumbled, under my breath. But I left Mom and crossed the hall to my room. I wished they'd send the baby back to the hospital where they got her. She didn't do anything but sleep, and everybody thought that was cute. They didn't watch me sleep.

Good Girls Don't

I crawled up on top of my bed, hung my head over the side and stared at the ceiling. I traced the clean white maze through the open door of my bedroom into the hallway and glimpsed the closed door where Mom slept with my new sister. I liked the way the closet doors suspended from the top, turning everything upside down. I had discovered this alternative view of my home while I was in bed for two weeks with the measles and learned to entertain myself walking on ceilings and stepping over tops of doors to enter rooms.

After a while Ruth called me from behind the closed door and invited me into Mom's room. She pulled up a rocking chair and told me to sit in it. "Hold her real carefully; never take your eyes off of her for a minute," she warned. "Never, ever touch the baby on the top of her head. The slightest touch can make a big hole right into her brain. This is where God finished her and sometimes there isn't quite enough to go around, so it takes longer to come together there," she explained.

Finally, she put Goldie into my arms and I looked into her face for the first time. Her eyes were squeezed shut and her mouth made comical puckering sounds. I examined her fingers and thought how different she felt from my dolls. She was warm and wriggly and made funny faces, kind of like the pet white mouse we kept in a cage at school. I sort of like her, I thought. I sang *Rock-a-Bye Baby* to her all the way through to the end.

"Hi Goldie, I'm your big sister," I whispered, the emphasis on big. "You can let me know if there's anything you need. Mommy's tired now so I'll be in charge," I said with authority.

I secretly wished she'd come a little older. What I really meant when I asked for a brother or sister was someone who played jacks or jump-roped or at least could talk. Since she did none of these things I realized I'd have to wait until she could be a pal. It would be a long time before the seven-year gap closed and I no longer had to wait.

As one might imagine, Goldie was a beautiful baby. Her now-famous enormous blue eyes and blonde ringlets challenged anyone, even then, not to fall in love with her. Golden from the beginning, she never had to grow into her name. It was impossible not to look at her.

CHAPTER 4

NO MATTER HOW MANY SPECTACULAR ADVENTURES or surprises life deals you, those moments that surround the beginning of first love stay with you, young and infinitely detailed.

I was a high-school sophomore in the fifties and wanted nothing more in life than to be 18, or at least 16. I had straight red hair — not auburn or strawberry or henna, but crimson red. There was hardly a hint of curve to my torso and I was convinced that no boy would ever look at me.

Takoma Park, Maryland, which is located directly north of the district line of Washington, D.C, was a little town whose identity was slightly blurred as a result of its close proximity to our nation's capital. It was, however, a bona-fide small town, replete with its own rendition of Main Street, though we called ours Carroll Avenue. Lining this avenue were Packet's Drug Store, Laurel Market, the Takoma Theater, Roberta's Ballet School and Hawn's Jewelers, which happened to be owned by my parents. As with many a small town, the bulk of Takoma Park's day-to-day business was done on this little strip. You couldn't walk down Carroll Avenue on a Saturday without bumping into someone you knew, a fact that was both comforting and irritating, depending on who you ran into.

Takoma Park was the kind of place that had four definite and distinct seasons, each of which was marked by its own particular ritual or event. Spring had officially sprung when the first azalea blooms began to pop open and saturate the air with their sweetly distinct odor. Part of growing up in Takoma Park meant a mandatory springtime visit to Piney Branch Road to see Mr. Pratt's azalea gardens. Summer was always heralded by lightning bugs and our annual Fourth of July parade, which began sharply at 9 a.m. and ended in fireworks. Winter was characterized less by early Christmas decorations than by seeing mothers and fathers using their credit cards to scrape the first frost off their car windows. And fall was always ushered in by the rich red and gold of the changing leaves, and of course, the start of school.

In the fall of 1956, Montgomery Blair High School was the focal point of my existence. At the center of my intellectual life was my body's refusal to comply with my ardent desire for maturity. Unlike most of my friends who had already begun to fill out and move on from their training bras, my budding breasts seemed content to remain confined to the triple-A cup my mother bought for me more out of compassion than necessity. Nor did my slim, boyish figure show any signs of widening at the hips, as the bodies of so many of my friends had done. I was the youngest kid in my neighborhood, and looked every bit the part. And like most kids, I wanted nothing more than to fit in.

Which is how, on the morning of my first day of high school, I found myself noiselessly creeping into Mom's closet, searching through her "party clothes" for something that would give me the lift I need. I was used to the smell of heavy Fabergé perfume mingled with stale cigarettes that filled the closet as I looked for her green satin dress. I knew she hadn't worn it in ages, so I snipped out the shoulder pads with cuticle scissors. I knew I was taking a chance but I was desperate. I tiptoed over to Daddy's closet and reached inside the pocket of his tuxedo pants to pull out a quarter and dime, which bought my lunch at school.

"How much are you taking?" Daddy asked, as he did every morning, eyes still closed.

"Thirty-five cents," I whispered.

Daddy's long black socks lay coiled on the hardwood floor beside his twin bed, looking a little dangerous. As usual, Mom, who slept curled up inside of herself on her own bed like a cold kitten, showed no sign of hearing our exchange.

I returned to my bedroom with the shoulder pads, which I placed inside my bra, added a couple of my own half slips and layered them under my skirt for hips until I was satisfied I looked at least 16. I slid my hands over my newly rounded curves and practiced walking in front of the mirror.

But my confidence quickly dissipated the moment I met up with my friend Patsy at the corner.

"You look funny," she said, eyeing me suspiciously, "Are you wearing falsies?"

"No," I lied. "It must be the new sweater. I think it's too tight."

"Why are you walking like that, then?"

I could see she wasn't going to let me off the hook, so I ended up telling her my underwear secrets in quiet, furtive whispers, even though there was no chance of being overheard.

"Do I look really weird?"

Patsy was a good friend. Though she was three years older, she always looked out for me, like an older sister. She might act bossy sometimes, but she wouldn't hurt my feelings for the world.

"No. You look OK," she said reassuringly. "Just don't stick your chest out so much when you walk."

We made it to the bus stop just in time and chose a seat in the middle section. I concentrated on looking older — affecting the elegant walk of the models I'd seen in the movies, who skimmed down runways as if walking on air. Then suddenly, a loud voice echoed forth from the back of the bus, smacking me in the face.

"Patti Hawn has falsies on! Patti Hawn has falsies on!"

The voice droned on in a singsong lilt; then finally the bus was deadly quiet. I knew the voice belonged to Jack Cotton, the class bully. Jack and I had gone all through elementary school together. We had a history, Jack and I. There'd been an incident in the fourth grade involving my lunch money, which Jack had stolen and put on the railroad tracks as a "science experiment." When Mom found out, she was so incensed that she called Jack's mother, who grounded him for the next three weeks. I guess he never forgave me for telling on him, because he seemed to be taking immeasurable pleasure in my discomfort at this moment. Jack was one of those kids who grew so fast he was heads taller than anyone in the class. His arms and legs looked like they belonged on another body. We called him Jack the Human Beanstalk.

We continued the ride to school in silence. I would not let the tears welling up inside my throat reach my eyes. I pictured Jack being run over by a diesel truck that passed us on the road. To keep the tears from falling I imagined how he'd look with his long beanstalk arms and legs scattered over the highway. Patsy slipped her hand over mine and squeezed it, and I wanted to cry more, so I just stared straight ahead, still feeling everyone's eyes on me. How could I make the shoulder pads disappear before we got to school?

The bus pulled up to the school parking lot. Patsy joined a group of her friends from the previous year, moving with the sophisticated grace of someone who had done this before. Though we had been friends for many years, in school she ignored me. After all, she was a junior and I was only a freshman. But just this once, I wished I could break the rules and we could be friends here too.

Jack bumped up against me as he exited the bus and I nudged him back, trying to muster some confidence, something to give me momentum to get through the day. "You make me barf, you big old string bean," I muttered.

Jack just grinned and wandered off into the crowd of kids who swarmed around him, buzzing with first-day-of-school excitement. I wanted to be one of them.

High school lay before me like a space needing a story, like the empty three-ring notebook that I clutched to my chest as I followed the path through the large oak trees that led to the front of the school. It was September and the temperature was finally cooling down. One thing I really liked about Maryland was autumn. There was never a question of its arrival. One minute we were sipping lemonade and sitting in front of a table fan and the very next day a slight chill charged the air and the trees colors were turned up a notch. Sweaters magically appeared out of cedar chests and smoke curled from chimneys.

I put my head down and headed for the nearest girl's room to remove the shoulder pads from my bra — but instead I was halted by a pair of feet that stood directly in my way.

He wore a white shirt with rolled-up sleeves and khaki pants. A red and white letter sweater hung low off one shoulder and a cigarette rested defiantly in the side of his mouth. He had thick brown wavy hair and hazel eyes. But it was his curling smile that got me, a mixture of kindness and mischief.

"So the string bean makes you barf. Those are pretty big words for someone as little as you."

He was definitely not a freshman. I could tell by the easy way he leaned against the wall. He looked at least sixteen. I pressed the notebook hard against my chest. For a minute I could barely catch my breath, but I forced myself to act normally.

"Sometimes you just have to say what you think," I some-how managed to say.

"You're a feisty one," he responded, smiling. I like that."

He winked at me and dropped his cigarette to the ground, grinding it into the dirt as though he'd been doing it for years. I watched him as he turned and joined his friends walking into the auditorium.

The rest of the day I searched for a glimpse of him in the crowded halls and darted into the girls' room at every opportunity to rub lipstick on my cheeks and check myself in the mirror. All the moments of my life faded from view, cowering behind that moment that hadn't yet occurred, the moment when I'd see him again.

CHAPTER 5

I DROPPED MY BOOKS ONTO THE DINING ROOM TABLE, seeing at once that Daddy was already home. A stuffed pheasant, a wedding gift from my grandfather to my parents, sat perched on the mantle piece in our back room, staring at me through a pair of sunglasses. He also wore a long black hairpiece held in place by a silk headscarf that tied under his beak. I noticed this with only mild interest, as I'd grown used to such oddities in my house. It simply meant that Daddy had returned home late the previous night, tied one on and decided to add his own sense of style to my mother's decorating scheme. I learned early to read the previous night's events by the status of the pheasant, my barometer for the mood of the household.

The new wall phone in our kitchen rang and I grabbed a coke from the refrigerator before I answered, assuming it was Patsy calling to tell me to hurry up and come over.

"Hi. Is this the cute little redhead who hates string beans?"

Through my shock, I must have somehow indicated that it was, in fact, me, but I don't remember actually speaking.

"It's Robert. Remember me? I met you this morning, outside the auditorium."

"Sure, I remember. You were smoking a cigarette." My voice sounded like it belonged to someone else, as if I were eavesdropping on another conversation.

"Yeah, I just started to smoke," he said. "I really don't know how to do it very well yet." For just a moment his voice, a little too loud, a little too brave, dropped a notch. "So, would you like to go to the back-to-school dance with me on Friday night? I just got my driver's license and I can borrow my dad's car." His voice picked up, gaining confidence. "I'll fill you in on everything you need to know to be a freshman."

I looked down at the Coke in my hands. It was sweating almost as much as I was.

"How did you find me?"

"Oh, I get around," he said, lowering his voice. "I can find out pretty much anything I want to know if I want to know it badly enough."

Ten minutes later I was sitting on Patsy's front porch watching her eyes grow wide with disbelief. "Robert Marsden is one of the most popular boys in school! He's already gone steady with two girls and is running for president of the student council. I can't believe he asked you out."

Her utter shock was disarming. Why would someone like him be interested in me? Patsy must be thinking the same thing, because she looked surprised and said thoughtfully, "Well, we know one thing for sure. He must really like you to have gone through all the trouble of finding your number."

Somehow this only made me feel worse. He must have thought I was someone else and the minute we were alone together he'd realize his horrible mistake.

"I don't even know what to say to him. What are we gonna talk about?"

Patsy laughed. "You'll think of something; you always do."

Friday afternoon, out of breath, I took the stairs two at a time and yelled to Mom, who was in the kitchen, that I wasn't hungry. I didn't wait for her response but escaped into my bedroom and closed the door. Today had been a busy day for me. I'd taken my first biology test, followed by a bewildering geometry class, during which I received a note from my father saying that he needed me to fill in at our watch shop because he'd gotten an unexpected music job. Now it was five o'clock and I only had a few hours to get ready for the dance and my date with Robert. I felt seriously pressed for time. I quickly laid my yellow sweater set on the bed and hopped into the shower. I let the hot water pour down my face while I planned my big entrance. I imagined myself as Scarlett O'Hara swooping down the stairs in the scene where she first meets Rhett Butler.

The hot shower calmed my nerves a little. I wrapped my hair in a towel and wiped the fog off the mirror. I spent the next several minutes examining my face and trying out expressions. I attempted to smile so my gums wouldn't show, but realized this only accentuated the small gap between my front teeth. So I switched to smiling harder on my left side, which made my dimple more prominent. Only somewhat satisfied with my smile, I moved on to other features, scrutinizing each minor detail to see what could be improved. I soon realized that if I squinted my eyes, just so, they wouldn't take up quite so much room on my face. My pale lashes, on the other hand, were beyond help. I wished more than anything that they were long and dark. I tried lifting one eyebrow for a dramatic effect, but the hairs were so light it just looked like I'd gotten something in my eye. Fortunately my skin still remained slightly tanned from the summer sun, which gave me a little more color than usual. I sighed. It was the best I could do for now.

I sat on the edge of the toilet carefully pulling nylons over my thighs and fastened them to the slender garter belt that circled my waist. I dropped a pink slip over my boyish body and sprayed lilac-scented toilet water around my face. After I pulled the sweater over my head and combed though my long red hair, I carefully closed the clasp on the single strand of pearls that my parents gave me for my thirteenth birthday. I stared at my reflection. I guess I'm not hopelessly ugly, I thought, but I'm no beauty either. I guess I fit somewhere in the middle.

I checked the time and realized that Robert would be arriving any minute. I quickly slipped into my parents' dark bedroom and found a spot behind the curtain where I had an unobstructed view of the street. After a few minutes I saw headlights pull into our driveway and was suddenly seized with panic. I watched Robert hop out of his father's green Chevrolet and stride over to our porch. From this distance I could see that the sleeves of his white shirt were rolled up above his elbows and his khakis neatly pressed, but I couldn't see his face. I held my breath and began counting from the time he knocked on our door until my mother finally opened it. It took exactly sixty beats.

I moved my post to the top of the stairs where I could see the top of my mother's head as she opened the door. I heard Robert introduce himself and then I watched as my mother moved to the side a little to let him in. For a second, the glow from the front porch light slightly shadowed his face. But when he stepped into the light of the hallway, everything came into focus. He looked like a movie star.

"You must be Robert. Please come in," my mother said in her overly polite company voice. I hated that fake voice. She sounded like one of those ladies on television who sold refrigerators. "It's a pleasure to meet you. Have a seat; Patti should be down in a minute." Her words all ran together as if she, too, had been practicing. She called for me to come down but I pretended not to hear. I wanted to appear as though I'd been otherwise occupied instead

Good Girls Don't

of hanging around in the upstairs hallway. She called again, louder this time.

Finally, I began the descent down our stairway. The stairs curved toward the bottom, and I was so preoccupied with smiling that I didn't notice the pile of books I'd left on the edge of the steps earlier. My heel caught on my geometry book and I lost my balance, tumbling down the last three steps, falling into a heap. I cried out, in spite of myself, as I untangled from a twisted ankle and saw in horror that my ripped skirt exposed my thigh to the top of my stocking. My embarrassment outweighed the pain, but when I tugged at my skirt, it ripped even further. I squeezed my eyes together really hard so the tears would disappear. I didn't dare look up at Robert. Instead, I stared stupidly at the scattered strand of pearls broken in the fall.

Mom got to me first. She pulled me to my feet, her company voice quickly replaced by her more normal tone.

"Are you OK? Jesus Christ, Patti, I told you not to wear those shoes! You're going to kill yourself. Sit down and let me have a look at you."

I still couldn't' look at Robert, who, by this time, was standing next to my Mom mumbling something about hoping I was OK. I pulled myself away from Mom's grasp, gave her a warning look and arranged my face into an expression that suggested this whole horrible event had never taken place.

Although my ankle hurt I showed no sign of pain, and when at last I found the courage to look at Robert, I smiled as hard as I could, letting him know with a hidden roll of my eyes, that my mother was overreacting. I could barely believe it when he knelt down beside me and helped pick up the maze of pearls. We sat together on the floor, not speaking, and searched for the pearls. After a few moments he handed his collection to me, our cupped hands lightly touching. I felt electricity shoot through me. He must have felt something too, because I stole a glance at him and could see that he was looking at me. Mom's voice cut into our silence.

"Will you please leave the pearls; I'll get them later. Patti, go upstairs. Your stockings are ripped and you need to change that skirt."

When I returned to the living room my mother was smiling her really big smile, the one that showed off her perfectly even teeth, at something Robert had said. She blew cigarette smoke in long elegant puffs and balanced a glass ashtray on her knee. She'd brought out a baking dish with chunks of fudge cut into large squares and offered one to Robert, who gladly accepted. They looked so comfortable together that for a moment I was almost jealous. I could see now why Mom was always the life of the party. She had such an easy way about her. I made a noise to let them know I was there.

Robert and I didn't speak very much during the fifteen-minute ride to the school gym. I watched his profile from the corner of my eye as he easily shifted the car into second gear and turned a little knob attached to the steering wheel, his other arm casually draped on the open window. I pretended great interest in the passing houses of my neighborhood, all of which I saw every day of my life. Eventually, he broke the silence.

"I hope your ankle isn't hurt too much to dance."

"Oh no," I responded, too eagerly. "I hardly hurt myself at all. It just looked stupid." I felt the blood rushing to my face. I was glad it was dark outside so he couldn't see me blush.

"You didn't look stupid. Anybody would have tripped with all those books piled all over the stairs." Then he smiled at me, and my breath, trapped inside my chest since the fall, rushed out like wind.

Next morning, Patsy was at the front door before my eyes were open, but I didn't want to see her quite yet. If I awoke maybe

I'd find out the night before had never happened. I needed to get everything clear in my mind before I could face the day. I remembered a huge, foil-covered papier-mâché ball suspended from the center of the gym casting points of light onto the wall, and strips of red and white crepe paper swaying from the ceiling. I lingered over a memory of Robert's hand on my back, pushing me toward him so my head burrowed into the spot directly under his shoulder.

I heard Patsy running up the stairs, shouting "C'mon, get up, it's after nine. I can't wait to hear. How was it? Did he kiss you good night?"

I would tell her everything, of course, but I needed more time, just a moment more. I couldn't yet leave the dream. She pushed my door open, pulled the covers from around my head and gently shook me. When I still pretended to be asleep, she jumped in beside me, her words tumbling onto the bed like they used to when we played monopoly and she was winning.

"I've been waiting all morning to hear. Tell me from the beginning. Don't leave anything out. Is he a good kisser?"

I hadn't a clue what a good kisser was supposed to do but I figured Robert must have done it right. When he dropped me off at the front door and leaned down to say good night, he pressed his lips hard against mine and his mouth opened a little. I wasn't sure what I was supposed to do but I definitely wanted to get it right so I put my hand behind his neck and gently rubbed the back of his hair like I'd seen Deborah Kerr do to Burt Lancaster in *From Here To Eternity.*

I rolled over to my back and sunk into the large feather pillow looking dreamily up into my friend's impatient face.

"It was the most perfect night of my entire life. There's absolutely nothing I would change about it. Even the part where I fell down the steps and thought I'd broken my leg and he ran across the room and picked me up in his arms and laid me on the couch." I paused for dramatic effect, stealing a sideways glance at Patsy to make sure she was impressed. Patsy, who by this time was lying on her side, her head propped up on her arm, shifted, and looked directly at me.

"He did what?" Her eyes narrowed. "You didn't break your leg. For crying out loud, Patti, can't you just tell me what happened? Why do you always have to make stuff different than it is?"

"Well, maybe he didn't pick me up, at least not right away, but I definitely fell down the stairs. And I don't make stuff up. I just exaggerate sometimes. There's nothing wrong with that, it just makes things more interesting."

"I saw you dancing with him. Everyone noticed. Even Jackie DiMaggio said something. And you know who she is."

Everyone knew Jackie DiMaggio. She was the most popular girl in school: a pretty, large-breasted cheerleader who everyone knew wore her sweaters too small, without a slip. She liked showing off her chest, sometimes even revealing her nipples if it was cold enough. People came not only to watch football but also to see if it was cold enough to get a look at Jackie's nipples.

"What did she say?" I asked, astonished. "Does she know my name?"

"Of course she doesn't know your name; you're just a freshman. Don't be stupid. But she knows Robert's name, that's for sure," she added slyly. "He went steady with her last year for a month. Even gave her his class ring."

"Why did they break up?"

"Nobody could figure it out. They seemed like the perfect couple. He was president of the class and she was a cheerleader. They just seemed to go together. I think she liked somebody else because she's had lots of boyfriends since."

This is not the conversation I wanted to have. I didn't want to hear about Robert with Jackie DiMaggio or anybody else. Who cares if she was older with big boobs, and popular? He wasn't dancing with her last night. He was with me. Nat King Cole wasn't singing to her. Those words were only for us. He loved me, I could tell. He probably wanted to marry me someday or at least give me his class ring. And I wouldn't ever give it back like Jackie did. Not ever.

"How does he kiss?" Patsy changed the subject.

"Kind of like Burt Lancaster."

"Did you let him French-kiss you?"

"Sure," I shrugged. "We did that twice."

She paused, seemed impressed. "You better be careful he doesn't think you're cheap. Kissing is fine but not on the first date. And French-kissing can get dangerous."

By this time we were both under the covers, our voices were soft, almost whispers.

"Patsy, promise you'll never tell anyone what I'm going to say, not anyone." I added, leaning forward toward her, almost touching, "and you can't laugh."

"I promise," she answered respectfully.

"Does French-kissing mean he puts his tongue in your mouth?"

"Yes," she said, slightly condescending. "You probably should only let him do that if he says he loves you."

"What do you do with your tongue?" I asked.

"Well, you touch tongues a little," she said. "Just not too much."

"I was lying when I said we did it twice," I admitted. "He just opened his mouth a little, but I never felt his tongue. I swear. Give me your arm and I'll show you what it was like."

Patsy rolled onto her back, not looking at me, and threw her arm over my chest in an act of exaggerated disdain. "If you ever tell anyone I let you do this I'll never speak to you again."

I pressed her forearm against my slightly open mouth, making certain my tongue was safely pressed against my bottom teeth, out of danger. I pressed so hard I left a tiny drop of saliva on her skin. She screamed in mock horror.

"Yuck, look what you did! You got spit all over me." She yanked her arm away from my mouth, rubbing it on the crisp white sheet, leaving a spot. "You better not do that to him or you'll never get a boyfriend," she giggled.

"I already have one, and he's going to marry me."

After a while, we were laughing so loud, doubled up on the bed, falling into each other's arms, that Goldie, who'd been instructed to never open my door without knocking, barged in.

"Sissy's getting married," she chanted, "and I'm telling Mom."

The following Monday at school, Robert was waiting for me when I get off the bus. He was wearing a moss-green sweater that matched his eyes and for a moment, when he saw me, I forgot I wasn't beautiful. He was standing with a couple of friends, but quickly walked toward me, yelling loudly over his shoulder, "There's a cute little redhead I've gotta go see over there." He looked really hard into my face and broke into a grin and laughed, "Has anyone ever told you how cute you are? I don't know whether to send you to camp or ask you on a date."

With one fluid motion he placed my hand inside of his and led me up the walkway past the groups of kids standing around waiting for the bell to ring. My hand trembled inside of his, so he held it tighter. I felt something flutter deep inside my belly I'd never felt before.

At sixteen Robert was already six feet tall. His face, full and boyish, still held traces of the child he was, but his shoulders were broad and looked almost as though they'd grown ahead of him. He fit inside his body like someone comfortable with being

Good Girls Don't

noticed. Not arrogant, just aware of himself. As a sophomore he had won the leading role in the senior play, *The Hasty Heart*, playing a young Scotsman who learned he was going to die. The part called for the actor to wear kilts on stage, which limited his competition among the 10th-grade boys, but Robert made a joke about it and wore them like he'd just come off the highlands. After that he became president of the theater club and appeared in all the school plays. His popularity in high school was sealed after his appearance as the roguish Billy, in the musical *Carousel*.

High school popularity was a rare and privileged state of the highest order whose members were entitled to certain indisputable favors, the most important of which was belonging. I'm sure they never knew where or to whom they belonged, but once established, that belonging was a state from which it was almost impossible to fall. To be popular was to be whispered about in reverence and treated with respect. Robert was popular. Unfortunately, I was not.

CHAPTER 6

BY EARLY DECEMBER, JUST OVER TWO MONTHS since Robert and I began dating, winter cold replaced the autumn chill and I could barely remember a time before him. When weren't together I waited for his phone calls. When we were together I waited to be touched. When I returned home I lay awake reliving the moment inside his parked car where he first told me he loved me.

Fine snow sprinkled the night sky like powdered sugar. The tops of the trees were barely visible from inside the 1941 Chevy. We watched snow fill the windows with sheets of thick frosting, blocking everything except the light from the car radio. Robert leaned over and adjusted the heater as I scanned the stations, settling on Tony Bennett singing *Because of You*, my favorite. I sang along with Tony, making my voice quiver a little during the part where he said "forever and ever." I watched Robert's arm, his hand just a silhouette against the radio's red light, and felt its pressure as he pulled me toward him so that my cheek rested against his rough wool jacket. When the song was over I reached into the warm bag lying on the seat between us, pulled out a French fry and held it out to him. He opened his mouth, allowing me to push it in, and clamped his lips around my fingers. Catsup smeared his mouth, dripping on his chin, and we laughed as I attempted to clean him with a napkin. Awkward, for just a moment, I licked my finger and looked away. When we were clean again he reached into his pocket, removed a small object and placed it into my palm. I clenched my fingers around the metal object, afraid to look.

"It's my class ring," he said, leaning over to kiss me. "Will you go steady with me?"

The snow had almost reached the top of the window, blocking all light except for a slit at the top. I could no longer see him, only feel his breath against my ear.

"Yes," I whispered. "I will." The large ring cut into my hand, but I didn't feel anything except the scratchy fabric of his coat against my face. I tilted my head, waiting for his lips that tasted salty from fries and smelled faintly of catsup and cigarettes. He opened my hand, took the ring and placed it on my finger, but it was so big it fell onto my lap. For the first time I saw it, through the sliver of remaining light. It was a wide gold band with a slightly raised black monogram displaying MB, the Montgomery Blair insignia, in large letters.

Robert pressed his palm up against mine, comparing our hands. His were twice the size of mine; my little finger ended where his began. He found my mouth again, only this time I kissed him back, holding my lips against his longer than usual. He drew me into his arms, easing me down into the seat until I was lying with my head propped up on the corner of the door. He pulled his face away to look at me in the dim light to see if I'd look back, and when I did, he kissed me again, slipping his hand underneath my coat skimming my breast. I grabbed his hand, as I knew I should, as I had been taught, and pushed it toward my shoulder—but the warmth in my stomach had already begun to spread along my thighs. He kissed me again, this time shifting his body directly over me. I felt his leg drop over mine, between my legs, awakening an exquisite urgency buried somewhere deep. We both breathed fast—in rhythm. My mouth filled with his and I shivered, even though I was warm. In one movement his hand reached under my coat, unbuttoned my cotton blouse, and pushed up my bra. He covered my small breast with his hand as though somehow this would protect it from danger. When he put his mouth on my nipple I sank into the warmth that streamed through me.

"I love you," he whispered into my ear.

And I believed him. I felt him tremble against me as I spoke his name and caressed his face, gently moving him away.

"I can't, we have to stop."

"I know," he said, pulling away. "I won't ever hurt you."

We lay breathing together, side-by-side, in the dark car, without moving. He shifted his body, which awkwardly pressed my head against his chest. My neck was pulled and it was hard to breathe, but I didn't move or utter a sound. I was afraid he'd turn away if I did. The windows of the car were steamed over so we could no longer see the snow.

Finally, he sat up and made a motion to leave. I turned away from him, pulled my coat around me and buttoned my blouse, quickly hiding myself, as best I could. The ring had fallen to the floor of the car and I swooped it greedily into my palm and buried it in my coat pocket, to be scrutinized later.

"We have to get you home," he said. "You won't be allowed to see me anymore and we can't have that." I like the way he said "we." Nobody had ever referred to me as a "we." It sounded grown up—so safe.

I knew Mom would be awake but I didn't want to see her. She'd be in the back room waiting to hear about my date. She liked to hear about what everyone had worn and who was going with who and what the parents of my friends were like, but I didn't want to talk to her tonight. I wanted only to crawl into my bed and re-live every second of the evening. I didn't want to ever forget it. I'd show her the ring tomorrow.

I lay on my bed and wondered what I'd be like when I became a woman. Surely by then I'd know what it's like to go all the way. I hoped I wouldn't have to wait until I was 20 or 21. I couldn't imagine being a virgin for that long.

I slipped under the sheets and raised my flannel nightgown under my chin and cupped my breasts. They felt a little like the mosquito bites I got every summer that swelled up after I'd scratched them too much. I tried to push them together to see if I could create the illusion of cleavage, but they barely budged. I wished they looked like Mom's. Hers were really big. I laid one hand sideways across my belly and easily touched my hipbones. I let my hand rest on the soft down between my legs that had recently begun to feel like velvety moss. I tried to imagine what it must feel like to have someone buried deep inside my body. Maybe the atomic bomb would drop on Takoma Park and Robert and I would be the only two people left in the world and we'd have to do it or die. Or I could be told I had leukemia with only six months to live; nobody would think I was cheap if I did it then. Nancy Morrison, a girl in my school, ran off and married a sailor she met at the roller skating rink when she was only 15. I never talked to her about it, but Patsy said she definitely looked different afterwards. She walked slower and smiled as though she had a secret. I wanted more than anything to know this secret. I thought of little else.

Most of what I knew about sex I'd learned from books, novels passed around by girlfriends. Although Mom never really talked about it she didn't seem to care what I read. Daddy, however, was a different story. He never said anything to me, but if I forgot to hide the book I was reading, it would disappear.

I was reading a lot of steamy novels by Frank Yerby about plantation owners in the South who sneaked into the cabins of beautiful slave girls and pleased them with "throbbing members" and "nights of unspeakable ecstasy." I never did ask Daddy about the books, but I usually found them stuffed into the back of his closet with the covers torn off. Daddy must've thought that if a book didn't have a cover it was somehow safe. I'd pull them out from behind his white shirts on a shelf where Mom stacked his socks and boxer shorts. We never spoke of this to each other but played this game for a long time.

Daddy never directly reprimanded or corrected me about much. He acted through Mom, blaming her for my indiscretions. He hated lipstick, for example, and kept a box of tissues by the front door, silently handing me one before I left the house, or telling her during one of their late night battles that she'd better "watch her more carefully" and "why aren't her grades better in math?" Although Daddy was an artist, he rarely encouraged me to participate in the arts. To him, excelling in math and science were the keys to a good life. I could hear them arguing about me long after I'd gone to bed.

"She's a good kid," Mom would say.

"Well, just tell her to keep her legs crossed," he'd reply.

Although Mom talked volumes about everything from why Catholicism was ruining our country to how ballet should be danced, she rarely mentioned sex except to say, "Don't do it!" I once asked her if people ever did it at any other time than when they wanted kids and she said, "occasionally, I guess," and then dove into a long discourse on how sex can ruin your life.

"Always remember what I'm telling you: boys will always try to get you to do it, but if you do they'll never, ever respect you. And without respect you have nothing." She usually repeated "nothing" a couple of times. "A girl has only one thing to give and that's her reputation. Without that she's doomed."

Mom's penchant for drama was always at its best during the sex talks. She loved Goldie and me with a fierceness that exceeded her feelings about almost everything else in her life, and I suppose she saw sex—or boys, perhaps—as one of the main threats to our happiness. She lived for and sometimes through us, ready to protect us from any and all suspected dangers. Mom had lost her first born child to an unexplained death before I was born. She apparently discovered his tiny body one morning when he was three months old, lying in his crib. I suppose losing an infant child through something so horrific as this and the loss of her own mother at three years old were good enough reasons to want to keep a close eye on those she loved.

Her intolerance for our pain often took strange turns. Once when my sister was about a year old she tumbled out of her high chair onto the kitchen floor. She was unhurt except for a few scratches, but it upset Mom so much she grabbed the high chair and threw it down the cellar steps breaking it into pieces. When I was 10 years old, Daddy, against Mom's wishes, bought me a two-wheel bicycle for Christmas. I began to suspect something was up when I routinely found a flat tire whenever I wanted to ride it. I spent more time fixing the tires than I ever did riding the bike. It wasn't until years later that I found out Mom regularly took the air out of the tires after I left for school. It was her way of keeping me safe.

After that night in the car with Robert, everything changed. His class ring became my passport out of ninth grade obscurity into the elite society of high-school cliques. I became a member of Robert's crowd, receiving either girlfriend or mascot status; it was hard to tell which.

The following Friday night we went to a party at Dan

Elliott's house. He was Robert's' best friend; they'd known each other since third grade. Dan, a slight boy with frequently combed blonde hair parted on the side, wore thick tortoise-shell glasses and had a reputation for being one of the best dancers in Robert's crowd. He was going steady with Janie Barlow, so we spent a lot of time double dating with them. Janie wasn't the brightest girl in school but she was a cheerleader, small and curvy, and she laughed a lot. Boys really liked her, so I tried to copy everything she did. If she laughed at something, I laughed louder and longer. When Janie complained of cramps because she had the curse I had them too, only worse, and when she and Dan made out in the back seat at the drive-in, I'd watch her in the rear view mirror to see how far she let Dan go.

Dan's parents were gone for the evening, so six packs of beer, hidden earlier in the bushes outside of the house, were retrieved, and slow dancing replaced the earlier sounds of *Come On-A My House*. Someone turned the lights down so low it was hard to tell if kids were dancing or making out. Couples quietly paired off, sinking into corners of the rec room, forming clusters of bobbing heads. A silhouette resembling Siamese twins dance against the wall to Tony Bennett crooning *Blue Velvet* from a tinny portable 45-rpm record player on the floor.

Robert whispered for me to follow him upstairs where we could have some privacy, because he had something to tell me. I nodded and followed. My heart was racing. Maybe he was going to tell me something I didn't want to hear. I touched his class ring that now hung around my neck on a silver chain. We climbed the short stairway from the basement recreation room, entering the living room of the split-level tract house where Dan lived, and I felt I'd walked into somewhere I didn't belong. I hesitated, but Robert pulled my hand, assuring me it was all right. I couldn't imagine why he'd brought me up here.

Good Girls Don't

"Please, God, don't let him ask for the ring back." My prayer was simple, straightforward. "Don't let him break up with me, not yet."

"I know Dan's parents; they'll be out half the night. They've gone to the Chesapeake Bay to play slot machines. That means they won't be home for hours," Robert said, confidently guiding me through this house as if it was his own.

He led me into a room with a bed larger than any I'd ever seen. It was covered with a shiny pink bedspread that looked like a satin ball gown. Two matching pillows covered in the same shiny material were propped up against the headboard. Hanging behind the bed, a gold leaf reflected plastic red roses in a vase on the double dresser. Spotless white wall-to-wall carpet sank under my feet.

"Take your shoes off, " Robert commanded. "I think she dusts this place for fingerprints. I'm surprised she hasn't put a velvet rope around it. Dan's mother's sort of a nut."

I immediately removed my scruffy brown and white saddle shoes and placed them beside the door. Although I'd polished them earlier that day, they looked dirty in this room. I felt embarrassed—sort of like the time I walked in on my parents in the kitchen while Daddy was drinking, and he was holding a sausage against his crotch. Mom was laughing until they saw me and I pretended I didn't notice the sausage. Just like I pretended it was OK to be in Dan's parents' bedroom. Pictures that looked like stick figures drawn with black crayon hung on the gold brocade wallpaper, and a white translucent figurine of two naked people wrapped around each other and lit from the inside, stood on a pedestal in the corner. I was careful not to look at it too long.

Robert removed his loafers and casually threw them on the carpet. He sauntered over to the statue of the entwined lovers and turned a switch that sent blue lights shooting through the couple, making them look a little like miniature ghosts.

"Pretty neat, don't you think? Makes you wonder what goes on in here." I knew he was smiling even though I couldn't see his face.

"Yeah, it sure does." I tried to sound like being here was no big deal, but I really wanted to leave. I knew I was trespassing and it felt dangerous. I want to be back downstairs with Janie and Dan listening to Tony Bennett, snuggling in a corner, with Robert's arms around me.

Robert sat on the pink bedspread and motioned for me to join him. One of the pillows fell to the floor and when I ran over to try and put it back, he pulled me down beside him and kissed me. I kiss him back while my hand searched for the pillow. I wanted to put it back where it belonged.

"Leave that; we'll fix it later, " he said sharply.

"But what if they come back early?" My voice was small. He mustn't know I was scared. Janie wouldn't be scared. I bet she comes up here with Dan all the time. They probably laugh at the statue while they make out on the bed. Robert unbuttoned my rayon blouse, the one I had borrowed from Mom's closet. He deftly reached back with one hand and released my bra as I let the pillow fall to the floor. The slippery bedspread felt cool against my naked back.

Robert's voice abruptly changed into a husky, half-whisper, almost as though he was talking to an audience instead of me.

"I love you, Patti. You love me too, don't you?"

"Yes," I tried to imitate his sound, but my voice came out scratchy, like I was clearing my throat. "Yes, I do," I repeated, a little too loud. I smelled the Old Spice on his skin and felt him harden through his khakis. I thought this was how it must feel to be beautiful, like Mom. Lying on the bed felt different than the car. His hand reached underneath my skirt and lightly touched me through my panties. I let his hand stay there for a second, long enough to feel his fingers begin to push aside the elastic band of my thin cotton underwear, and I waited until the last moment to gently push his hand away.

I'd learned two new things about myself tonight. It was more thrilling to be desired than to desire—and I didn't like pink.

Mom was waiting up for me in the back room when Robert drove me home that night. She was reading a Pearl Buck novel, a clear sign that something was wrong.

For as long as I could remember, Mom had a few books she read over and over. If Daddy found comfort in sniffing horseradish, Mom found peace in Pearl Buck. A copy of *The Good Earth* held a prominent place on the bookshelf in our back room. I guessed this novel of peasant life in China in the 1920's created a perception of family that appealed to her, made her feel safe. Her other favorite book was *Heidi* and she re-read it at so many times during her life that the cover fell off.

I was not surprised to see the light in the back room. Mom often stayed up reading or watching television until I got home, but tonight she looked at me differently. I wanted to tell her I was still a good girl and hadn't done anything really bad, but it felt as though she looked right through me and knew I'd been on the big pink bed beside Robert.

She stood up when I walked into the room and dropped the book on the couch.

"He's too old for you," she began abruptly. Her voice was loud, accusing, and uttered as though it followed a list of other complaints.

"I don't like you running around with kids three years older. You're missing a huge part of your life, one you'll never get back. These kids are doing things you have no business being involved in. What does this boy see in you in the first place? You're much, much too young for him. I've heard you on the phone with him; you don't even sound like yourself. You put on a whole different voice for him and I don't like it. You're trying to keep up with a crowd that doesn't care a bit about you and I see nothing but trouble ahead. What the hell's wrong with the kids your own age? You don't see Judy Levine running around Takoma Park in high heels and lipstick." Her voice escalated.

"This going-steady business is for the birds. The only thing going steady is good for is taking Ex-Lax. Mrs. Cheek called me the other day and told me she saw you walk into the movie theater with bright red lipstick, high heels and earrings. She said you looked like a midget. I want you to stay out of my closet and you need to be home at a decent hour."

By this time she had come so close that I practically felt her spit spray on my face. "Your father, of course, never speaks to you, but he sure as hell complains to me. There's going to be some new rules around here." She got up from the couch, walked into the kitchen and never stopped talking. "Now go upstairs and wash that crap off your face and I expect you to help me around here tomorrow. We're going over to Ninny's on Sunday and I need you to help me clean the basement. Go to bed before your father gets home. I don't want to listen to any more of his complaints about you."

I said nothing but made my eyes look mean and scowled at her. "Don't give me any black looks. I'm your mother and you'll treat me with respect," she shouted.

"You can't make me stop seeing him," I whispered under my breath. "I'd die before that." I turned around and ran upstairs to my room. I won't let her see me cry, I vowed, under my breath. Out of sight, I whispered, "I hate you! You can't ever make me stop seeing him."

Good Girls Don't

I opened my bedroom door the next morning and heard Mom in her bedroom, whispering on the phone to Roberta.

"She stays in bed until noon, does nothing to help out around the house. She's quit dancing school. The only thing she can think about is this kid. He's too old for her, Bertie. This is going to come back and bite her in the ass, mark my words. She's stopped seeing all her friends and does nothing but lock herself up in her room and wait for him to call. Rut, as usual, won't deal with anything — so like always, I have to be the bad one. Where did she get such a mouth on her?! And you should see the black looks. You know all I want is the best for her but…"

I couldn't hear anything else but by the time I came downstairs she was quiet.

When Mom got mad she often took it out on inanimate objects. A cup was not placed on a table; it was hammered, like an exclamation point. Her small hands flew in a hundred directions, a language all to themselves.

"Sit down and eat, I made eggs and cream cheese." The dish hit the table in front of me like it had fallen from the ceiling.

"I need you to help me sweep the water out of the basement. It rained last night and the cellar is filled up again so get a broom after you finish and come down and help me."

By the time I got to the basement Mom had already moved large boxes of old clothes out into the yard and pulled the washing machine away from the wall; she had stacked an old metal kitchen table on top of the washing machine and was about ready to throw Daddy's fishing boots and Goldie's baby crib into a growing pile in the back yard.

"This Goddamned house is falling apart." She didn't yet see me and was talking out loud to herself. She pitched Daddy's old fishing rod on top of the heap with such force it bounced off the pile and landed on the ground.

"Does anybody ever help around here? I need this aggravation like I need another head. They expect me to do everything. Now I have to lie in bed at night and listen for her to come home at midnight. Of course I never think of anything good," she continued talking into the air, as though she expected an answer. "All I see is her laying under a car somewhere."

The pile grew bigger as Mom yanked the bricks away from the cellar wall she'd been saving for a fireplace she planned to build in the backyard. I wasn't sure what to do, but I grabbed a broom and started sweeping the water that had seeped underneath the basement door and now covered much of the cement floor.

"Don't use that broom," she yelled. "For Christ sake, Patti, use your head. We'll be here until the Thursday after never. Get the one in the closet."

I returned upstairs to get the larger broom and by the time I returned she had removed most of the contents of our basement and was standing with her hands on her hips staring into the pyramid of used up household belongings, her dark eyes blazing.

"You know, Patti, youth only happens once. You never get to do it again. It's a sin to waste a moment of it because it's probably the happiest you'll ever be in your lifetime — and you're skipping over a big chunk of it. I'm telling you this, and you'd better listen carefully: don't miss a minute of it; you'll never get it back — never."

"But Mom, I love him and he loves me," I pleaded. "I don't want anything else."

"Love!" by this time she's screaming. "Do you think you know anything at all about love? For Christ sake, Patti, you're fifteen years old, you don't know anything about anything."

"I know more than you think," I shouted, throwing the broom on the floor, running up the stairs.

Good Girls Don't

I ran across the street in back of Mrs. Harmon's house to Sligo Creek, to a secret spot I'd discovered when I was eight years old playing "explorer" with a neighbor kid. I collapsed in a heap among the oak roots that extended over the creek, creating a tangled seat. I scowled fiercely into the water. Either in my head or out loud—I'm not sure which—I heard the words, "I'll never leave him. I'll never leave him."

CHAPTER 7

WHEN THE CAB DRIVER DROPPED MOM, GOLDIE AND ME off at Ninny's the next day I felt a surge of relief. I entered into the warmth of stuffed cabbage and Uncle Charlie's tobacco, and saw Ninny in the kitchen from the front door. Her apron, stained with tomato splotches, hung from her neck. Heat from the stove made her thick white hair stick out in wiry spikes around her face.

I walked over and took my place beside her. She never once took her eyes from the stove as she stood over a large steaming pot, holding a big wooden spoon to her lips. She changed her mind mid-way, blew softly on the spoon and put the tangy tomato soaked cabbage into my mouth.

"Good!" she says, seemingly unaware I'd only just arrived.

"Maybe a little pepper."

"Pepper! – There's no pepper in this house. Your mother uses pepper. I don't. You never learned pepper from me. She probably puts pepper on her cottage cheese and canned pears." Ninny usually sounded a little mad about something, but it's the kind of mad you know isn't real.

Mom, who'd entered the kitchen by now, pushed a huge billowy cake to the center of the table.

Good Girls Don't

"Look, Tanta, I made the lemon cake with pudding this time. I saw it in *Better Homes and Gardens* — tastes entirely different."

"Hmm!" Although Ninny's sounds filled up rooms and spoke volumes, I was never sure if they were disapproving or just skeptical. But they definitely commanded my attention. My family spent absolutely no time on formal salutations. We did not knock on doors, say hello, good-bye or how are you. We kissed babies and each other at funerals and never said I love you. These gestures were looked upon as completely unnecessary acts of formality and usually, upon entering each other's homes, we dove directly into whatever was going on without ever missing a beat.

Ninny was my Aunt Sarah, sister to Aunt Goldie, but I always thought of her as my own grandmother. She and Uncle Charlie moved from Pittsburgh to Washington at about the time I was born. She was for all practical purposes my grandmother. I can never remember a time before her. If there was one unalterable constant in my life, it was Ninny. And there was never a question of who her favorite was.

My earliest memories were of Friday afternoons in the row house on Madison Street. I loved watching her set up the ironing board on the back porch. She always ironed on Fridays. I would sit at the kitchen table snapping green beans for Friday night dinner and watch Ninny dip her hands into a bowl of water and flick it on Uncle Charlie's white shirt until it was damp enough to roll up into a ball and stack at the end of the ironing board. I loved the part where Ninny spit on her finger and touched the hot iron to make sure it was the right temperature. I remembered thinking that she was the bravest person I knew. I watched with fascination as she chose a shirt from the stack of sprinkled clothes and spread it out on the ironing board. She always began with the collar.

Ninny would pause now and then to glance at a photograph on the bookshelf of a handsome young soldier and let out a significant sigh. A warm breeze might come in through the screen door and lift the white eyelet curtains from the window. The room would fill with Friday smells of roast chicken, damp clothes and freshly mowed grass from Mr. Green's lawn mower next door.

"Ninny, Fridays are my favorite day. I wish I could stay here with you forever."

"That would make your parents really sad. You know we've talked about this before."

Sooner or later, Ninny would say something in the way of a preamble to a story of her youth. It was the moment I waited for. She might point at the radio and say in a dreamy voice, "This reminds me of when I was a little girl in Budapest." This was my cue to pour myself a glass of milk and tuck my legs under my skirt. This is how Fridays are supposed to be, I thought.

"I was on the way to your grandmother's wedding but I got lost in Gypsy Town," said Ninny, slipping into a dialect like no other—part Yiddish, part Hungarian and part her.

"I met a gypsy fiddle player who promised to teach me how to play if I came back the next day. He was a young man who played so beautifully I had to stop and listen. I'd never heard music like that. We became friends even though I never knew his name. I secretly returned every day even though Mom had forbidden me to go to that part of town. Can you believe I learned to play the violin from a dark, handsome gypsy man whose name I never knew!"

We were getting to my favorite part. Here Ninny always widened her eyes in disbelief, coming toward me and lowering her voice. "This was a very big secret for a little girl to keep, but your great grandmother never knew until we came to this country. Everyone was so shocked that I, little Sarah, could play such a difficult instrument. Nobody ever knew where I had learned."

On one of those occasions, at the end of her story, she carefully lifted the stacked shirts off the ledge to take them upstairs when the volume on the radio took on a life of its own. A deep voice filled the warm kitchen with an announcement that Franklin Delano Roosevelt has just died. I watched the clothes fall to the floor as she dropped into the kitchen chair and clutched her trembling hands between her knees. We sat staring at a spot on the oilcloth table covering until, finally, tears came and she began to cry. I stooped down to pick up the shirts but instead she snatched me onto her lap. She held me like this for a long time while we waited for Uncle Charlie to come home.

Today, however, my thoughts were of self-preservation. I left the kitchen when Mom entered. Today I wanted to stay as far away from her as possible. I knew she'd tell Ninny about Robert and I didn't want their words intruding on my thoughts. I went into the living room and lay down on the couch, pretending I had fallen asleep. Uncle Charlie had taken Goldie to the store for more of the orange soda and ginger ale that always sat on Ninny's dinner table. Ninny usually carried a half-filled glass of ginger ale with her during her day. She said it helped digestion and God forbid if she ran out. I curled up facing the back of the couch and closed my eyes really tight, hoping I wouldn't hear their discussion. Apparently I really did fall asleep, because loud voices from the kitchen woke me.

"You think you were a picnic, Laura? You're no different than your kid. You don't think you made my sister crazy with the boys and the hair and clothes? Nothing was ever good enough for you." Her questions, rhetorical, apparently required no answers. "You always thought you were special, with the fancy clothes your no-good father brought you. Never satisfied, always had a mouth on you bigger than anyone else's. She's just like you, headstrong and smart. So don't tell me about her. The more you yell, the worse it'll be. If you don't let up on her she could make you a very young grandmother. Girls do get in trouble, don't they?"

———————————

After that visit to Ninny's, Mom changed. She stopped complaining so much about Daddy and money and her life, and instead wanted to know everything about my new friends. She still wasn't exactly thrilled about Robert but she didn't seem as mad about everything as before. Daddy was never home. He played music jobs every week, and several nights during the week, which gave Mom plenty of time to concentrate on me. She managed Roberta's dancing school during the days but was always home in the evenings. Although our late-night talks in the back room continued, they started to sound different. It was almost like my friends became hers and she knew more about them than I did. For a while it seemed our house had become the official teen drop-in center.

When Patsy's mother, who was at least twenty years older than Mom, didn't understand why Patsy wanted to live away at college instead of commuting every day, Mom paid her a visit to make her understand that young girls need to feel independent. Or, when Larry and Susan, who'd been a couple since the seventh grade, broke up, it wasn't Susan's mother who she went to for comfort, it was mine. Mom loved her new role as den mother, and soon the all-night stories in the back room turned away from tales of family to the exploits of my friends. She analyzed why Bob Short wouldn't stay faithful to Nora if they didn't attend the same college. Or when Mitch McNalley got caught for drinking beer in the parking lot, Mom rationalized he was just having a rough time because his parents had split up. She clinched her role as a Mom to be trusted after Dan's mother reprimanded Janie for wearing her skirts too tight, and Mom imitated Mrs. Elliot's shaky voice, calling her a dried-up old biddy.

I felt confused. I loved all the attention, but Mom was definitely a hard act to follow.

One Friday night at an impromptu party, Mom pushed the furniture aside and rolled up the living room rug so we could dance. Mom was wearing a new plaid dress, her tiny waist cinched by a narrow black patent-leather belt. Dan was playing the piano and everyone sang *100 Bottles of Beer on the Wall* as loud as we could. We sure wouldn't sing that song at Patsy's house, but Mom was standing next to Dan singing louder than everyone. Her eyes were sparkling; she looked really happy. She was laughing so hard she spilled her coffee on the piano, which made everyone laugh even more. Janie ran to the kitchen for a dish towel, but Mom didn't seem to notice. Robert, who was standing in the middle of the group, laughed the loudest.

It was sort of like watching a movie. I liked seeing Mom happy; she didn't get a chance to be that way very often with Daddy, who was so introverted. She was always complaining about how Daddy never took her anywhere, and here she was, in her own house, having so much fun. I kind of wished she'd be happy with her own friends, though. I left the party, climbed upstairs and locked myself in the bathroom and sat on the closed toilet seat, just listening for a while. My stomach hurt and I wanted everyone to go away, even Robert. I stayed there for a long time, but when I returned downstairs they were still singing. They'd gotten down to ten bottles of beer on the wall and nobody had ever noticed I'd left.

CHAPTER 8

A WEEK BEFORE MY 16TH BIRTHDAY, Robert took me to a drive-in movie, which we saw very little of from the back seat of the car. We were playing our usual game of "you can touch me here, but not there, well, maybe there, but not for too long," when Patsy and Gordy Stewart, who were in the front seat giggling, sat up and announced they needed to leave.

"We haven't finished the movie; what's the rush?" I complained. "We want to go to the Hot Shoppe," they said.

It was only 9:30, an hour and a half before Patsy's curfew, when her mom always began flicking the porch light on and off.

"I'm expecting a call from Diane Dobson at 10:30 and I want to make sure I'm there." Patsy was unusually terse.

Diane Dobson was a year or so older than Patsy. When Patsy had begun making plans to go away to the University of Maryland next year, she and Diane decided to be roommates. I didn't know her very well but felt a little displaced by their friendship and more than annoyed by this last-minute announcement.

Robert nudged me, whispering that we could get his car and still save the night, so I nodded and didn't ask questions, but gave Patsy a look she pretended not to see. After Gordy had dropped us off in front of my house, Robert and I slipped into his car and headed off for Sligo Creek Park to find our usual spot, where the streetlights stopped and the moonlight began. It was March and cold had given away to soft warm night air --- the kind that smelled of lilacs.

I listened to Robert talk about his college plans — to join a fraternity and maybe try out for the University Theater. A fear began to tug at me that had recently become hard to ignore. He'd soon be attending college. I could barely comprehend the ninth grade, but the university was another planet. He talked often about his plans to study theater, his desire to travel, maybe become an officer in the Air Force. And I listened. Sometimes I listened so intently, so loudly, I was afraid I'd be heard. If he paused for a moment, I'd nod gravely. I chuckled at his jokes as though they were secrets only we shared. I offered encouraging remarks, like, "of course you are," or "why in the world wouldn't you," or "everybody knows you'd be able to do that." My role came naturally, easily, as though I had been born to it.

Finally he stopped talking and in one motion switched off the car motor and pulled me toward him. I knew how his mouth tasted and his shirt smelled. I anticipated feeling his hand moving under my bra and cupping my breast, allowing his tongue to linger. I awaited the heat that would begin in my belly and warm me from a spot deep inside. This is what I waited for. I loved to hear his breathing become loud, his body harden and press against me, wanting me, wanting me so much, he must surely love me.

Robert spoke and his tone was longing, beseeching. "I really want to go all the way with you, Patti. I love you. Let me really love you."

"You know I can't do that," I whispered. "I want to, but we have to wait. I'm so sorry, I know it's hard for you," I apologized.

I slipped away from his probing fingers with just a slight tilt of my body so that his hand barely grazed between my legs. I allowed my body to linger against his until the exact moment I felt his thighs moving between mine. I slid out from underneath him and began to push him away. I wanted his body to drift into mine but then I remembered what Mom had told me about how he wouldn't respect me, and for sure would break up with me, and I shoved him away, more forcefully this time.

Light filled the car, blinding me. It moved down my body, exposing my breasts. Robert reacted first. He recovered so smoothly that I was surprised.

"Good evening, Officer." He tucked in his shirt as he spoke to the faceless voice coming from outside the car.

"Step out and let me see your license, please." The light continued to rudely expose me. I squeezed my eyes shut and pushed my feet into the floor mat, wishing I could escape into the back of the car.

"Yes, sir," Robert answered, a smile in his voice. He sounded exactly right—contrite but not afraid.

"You kids need to move along. This isn't allowed here. You're looking for trouble if you stop along this road."

The light finally moved away from me and onto Robert's driver's license. The officer studied as though it was important. His face, outlined in the moonlight, was soft, young.

We were just leaving, sir."

"Well, see that you do."

One more wave of the light, this time on my face.

"You, girlie, are too young to be here. Get yourself home right now."

"O.K, I will," I mumbled, on the verge of tears. I looked down at my blouse, buttoned wrong, hanging crooked from my shoulders.

We drove home in silence. Robert left me quickly at the door an hour earlier than I was expected.

CHAPTER 9

I CHECKED MYSELF IN THE HALL MIRROR, wiped off my lipstick, and tucked in my blouse, before I moved into the back room where I knew Mom waited. I arranged my face into what I imagined to be a distant blank look, once removed from anything remotely revealing about my evening, and prepared myself for Mom's gossip about my friends. Goldie was spending the night with her best friend, Anne Marie, and Daddy was working a late job. Mom was curled up on the couch reading and barely looked up from her book when I walked into the room. She told me Patsy had been trying to call me.

"You'd better call her, even though it's late. She's already phoned three times in the past hour."

I used the phone upstairs in my parents' bedroom so Mom couldn't hear. Whatever Patsy wanted must be important. Maybe Gordy had broken up with her and she needed to talk. By the time I climbed the stairs to the bedroom I'd convinced myself this must be it, and I was secretly pleased she'd called me instead of Diane.

Recently I'd become the ear for my girlfriends, doling out sage and insightful counsel about the problems of love. I liked giving advice and did it on a moment's notice, going over any given problem repeatedly from every imaginable perspective. I'd learned how to adjust my voice in such a way as to inspire implicit trust. Mom often walked by my spot at the bottom of the stairs where our telephone sat and rolled her eyes during my therapy sessions. She began calling me "Dear Abby" and suggested that I start charging a fee for "such amazing wisdom."

I'd already begun to formulate what I'd tell Patsy when I began dialing. After all, Gordy was not going to be attending college. He's already said he'd be joining the Navy and he really wasn't her type. Patsy answered the phone on the first ring, like she'd been sitting on top of it.

"What's going on?" I began. "You really didn't think I was going to come home at 9:30, did you?"

She interrupted. "Shut up and listen to me. Something really, really bad has happened and I don't know what to do." Her voice was an urgent hiss; I had to listen hard to understand.

"I can't talk long," she said. "My mom's in the next room and she already suspects something, so you have to help."

"OK. Just tell me what's wrong."

"First you have to promise, I mean really promise to never tell anybody about this."

Of course I promise, now tell me what's going on," I plead.

"Diane got into trouble and she went to someone to help her get rid of it and now I think she might die and she has nowhere to go because she can't go home and I don't know what to do 'cause she's in a phone booth by the Takoma Theater and someone's got to help her. She can't go home."

Her words tumbled out so fast they all ran together, so it took a minute for me to digest what she'd said.

"What do you mean, she can't go home? She has to go home. If she's going to die she has to go home."

"She can't go home, Patti, her parents must never know about this. The guy's one of the teachers at the University. C'mon, help me think. We've got to help her."

I don't even know her, I thought. This is way over my head. But I'd been chosen to help and knew this was an honor. If I could figure out something for this girl to do, my place among this older crowd would be firmly established. Besides, maybe she really could die.

I heard Patsy's mom in the background: "Get off that phone, missy." Mrs. Weir always called Patsy "missy" when she was mad. "You've been tying up that phone line all night. It's eleven o'clock. Who on earth are you talking to?"

"The number in the phone booth is Randolph 7521," Patsy says. "Diane's waiting to hear back from me. I have to go. Call me."

I sat on Daddy's bed with the phone number crumpled in my hand for no more than thirty seconds. I imagined poor Diane standing alone in a phone booth bleeding to death. I ran downstairs and yelled for Mom before I reached the bottom step. I told her everything Patsy had told me, even the part about the college professor. Without a moment's hesitation, my mother flew into action. She grabbed the paper out of my shaking hands and went directly to the phone to dial it.

"Diane, this is Mrs. Hawn," she said, her voice crisp and commanding. "I'm Patti's mother. Answer me carefully. How bad are you bleeding? …Uh huh, OK, that's not too bad. Are you in pain? OK. How long ago did you do this? Stop crying and answer me." She motioned for me to get a pencil and paper out of the drawer and bring it to her.

"Put the phone down and go outside and look at the cross street where you're standing. Come back and tell me exactly what it says," she commanded. Mom never took her eyes off the phone and in a few seconds she was scribbling down Eastern and Carroll Avenues.

"I'm hanging up and calling the Yellow Cab Company to pick you up and bring you here. Do not leave the phone booth under any circumstances." Then, as an afterthought, she asked, "Do you have money?"

Mom clicked the receiver, never taking it away from her ear. She looked at me for the first time.

"Go upstairs in my dresser and get five dollars out of the bottom drawer," she said. Grateful for something to do, I took the stairs two at a time and heard Mom in the background talking to the dispatcher at the cab company.

"This is Mrs. Hawn, Jerry. I need you to do something for me. One of Patti's friends is in a phone booth by the Takoma Theater." She repeated the address, pronouncing the street names with exaggerated precision.

"I want her brought here." Although the Yellow Cab Company was more than familiar with our house, Mom always repeated the address and directions. "Number nine Cleveland Avenue: that's a dead-end street right off of Baltimore, the red brick semi-detached house on the left-hand side of the street. I'll pay the driver when he gets here." Mom overemphasized her words, almost like she was talking to someone with a disability.

"I need someone there as soon as possible. It's too late for her to be out alone. Do you understand me? OK, I'll be waiting."

Mom finally looked up from the phone.

"Who the hell is this girl and how do you know her?"

––––––––––––––––––

By the time the cab pulled up in front of the house, Mom had pulled the covers off of my bed and replaced them with an old rubber crib sheet that she'd found in the back of the linen closet. We worked without words, side by side, remaking the bed until Mom handed me the money to go out and pay the cab driver.

I saw Diane hunched into the corner of the cab looking scared. I'd seen her with Patsy a few times but had never spoken much to her. She was four years older than me, a college freshman and worlds apart.

The last time I had seen her was in Patsy's bedroom a couple of weeks ago, sitting on the bed surrounded by fashion magazines. They'd been going over their plans to live together in the dormitory at Maryland University, and since I could add nothing to this conversation, I didn't stay long. I was beginning to feel more and more left out of my best friend's life. Patsy, who always had a crowd of friends older than I, had never let that interfere with our friendship before, but Diane was different. I felt replaced. She was a college freshman who'd been "pinned" to a fraternity man. She drank mixed drinks and smoked and went to clubs downtown where there was live music. Tall and slender with short black curls that framed a perfectly oval face, Diane had skin like the cream at the top of the milk bottle before it's shook up. She used her hands a lot when she talked and her fingernails were polished bright red and filed into perfect ovals. She treated me, that afternoon, like a pesty little sister of Patsy's even though she knew I went steady with Robert Marsden. This astounding addition to my credentials had made little difference to her.

Tonight she looked very different. Her large dark eyes were red and watery from crying and her curls were hidden under a large green scarf tied under her chin, making her look like a refugee from a war poster. I gave the five dollars to the cab driver and she grabbed my hand as soon as she got out of the cab.

"Patti, I can't go home. My mother mustn't know about this, not ever." She seemed more worried about her mother finding out than about the blood leaving her body.

"Patsy said your Mom's real understanding and maybe she'd help me. Will she tell my mother? If she will, I have to go somewhere else." She stopped in the middle of the path to the front porch and looked at me like she was ready to bolt if I gave the wrong answer.

I told her Mom wouldn't tell anyone. Truthfully, I wasn't sure what Mom would do at any given time; she was so full of surprises these days. But I knew there was nowhere else for her to go so, I told her anything I thought would calm her and make her stay.

"My mother knows a lot about this kind of thing," I lied. "And my father won't be home until real late tonight so I'm sure Mom will figure something out. She's good in emergencies." This with my most reassuring voice.

Mom, who was already on the porch waiting, got right to the point. Her questions were terse and purposeful, like those of a nurse. She asked Diane questions about how long ago she'd done it and if the guy who did it used a catheter and stuff like that.

Diane poured out her story like she was in a confessional. She'd missed her period and gone to a doctor somewhere in Washington, who proclaimed her to be a couple of months pregnant. The professor, who was married, found a doctor who agreed to do it and they met him at a bar in Easton. Apparently the professor and the doctor drove her to a house somewhere on the edge of town and she was told to remove her panties and crawl up on his kitchen table. The doctor said the professor could stay and hold her hand. She said it didn't hurt much when he put a long thing like a knitting needle inside of her. She said she didn't look but saw newspapers all over the floor and the doctor told her to look at her boyfriend while he did it. She kept saying how much she loved the professor, but her parents would never let her be with him, and she knew he loved her too but it was "doomed from the beginning."

This was the only time Mom gave Diane one of her looks. It was the same kind of look Ninny gave. I was used to it, to but

Good Girls Don't

Diane didn't talk too much about the professor boyfriend after that. The doctor told her she'd probably start to bleed in about five hours and she should pass the fetus sometime during the night.

I wondered what a fetus looked like. We'd seen pictures during health class of babies in different stages, and the best image I could come up with was a tadpole.

Diane continued her story, saying that the professor couldn't stay with her afterwards and dropped her off in front of her house. She said he'd already risked so much for her that she didn't want him to know she couldn't return home. She walked to the theater, because she didn't know where else to go. It was dark and nobody would see her and she thought she could think better there. She told Mom she was starting to get bad cramps and had already gone through a couple of Super Kotex pads in the last hour or so.

Mom instructed her to call her mother and tell her she was spending the night and would be home in the morning. She said to tell her we'd all been sitting around talking and the time had gotten away from us. She'd been invited to stay over because Mr. Hawn, who was going to drive the girls home, wouldn't be home from his music job until the middle of the night, too late to take her home. Diane, who by this time was doubling over with cramps, did exactly as she was told.

Mom and I listened from the hall in silence while Diane talked to her mother. It was as though we were holding each other's breath. It occurred to me that—in this speechless, officious partnership—we had somehow discovered a place to connect.

Diane pulled one of Mom's cotton nightgowns over her head and crawled into my bed. By the time Mom had brought her up a cup of tea Diane was crying again.

"Thank you so much, Mrs. Hawn. I don't know what I'd have done without you. My mother would never understand anything like this."

Mom just nodded and didn't talk much. I sat on the edge of my bed and tried to think of something to say, but in the end I, too, just sat, waiting. I didn't know exactly what I waited for, but Mom came in every so often and told Diane to get up and look at the pad. She and Mom went into the bathroom together and closed the door. After an hour or so of this, Diane was exhausted and was looking up at the ceiling a lot. I held a washcloth on her forehead and Mom took the sanitary napkin from between her legs. She examined it intently before rushing it off to the bathroom. A blood-stain shaped like the state of Florida had seeped onto the white sheet and every time Diane kicked the covers off I looked out the window even though it was too dark to see anything.

The front door opened and the thud of Daddy's saxophone case hit the floor. Mom met him on the stairs and told him a friend of mine was spending the night and had become sick.

"It's probably something she ate," she explained. She urged him to go to bed and told him she'd be in later.

Mom returned to my bedroom and motioned for Diane to be quiet. We said nothing to each other. Diane's face was blotchy, her eyes swollen and red. She grabbed Mom's hand and squeezed it and looked up at her like my mother was some kind of saint. I again took up my vigil at the dark window and made up a poem that played in my head.

> *Diane, Diane, full of woe*
> *No where else for you to go*
> *My mother's hand is on your head*
> *You've stained her sheets a crimson red*

I felt oddly annoyed by this scene taking place in my bed-room. I knew I should feel sorry for Diane and I wanted to, but I really wished she'd gone to her own mother or grandmother or anybody but my mother. I didn't feel a part of what was going on,

Good Girls Don't

almost like I was a stranger in my own bedroom. Mom was acting like she was some kind of a doctor or something. I didn't know why it irritated me, especially since I was the one who had brought Diane here, but nobody had even looked at me. I wondered if Mom would hold my head like that if it were me in that bed instead of a stranger. I guess I knew she would. She'd probably be mad that I'd had sex with someone, but for sure she'd hold my head. I remembered how cool her hand felt on my forehead when I was sick and throwing up into the toilet. She always pressed hard and it helped. If I was really sick and couldn't make it to the bathroom she always told me not to worry, she'd clean it up later.

I fell asleep sometime during the night curled up at the bottom of my bed. When I awoke the following morning Diane was still asleep and Mom was with Daddy in their bedroom, like nothing had happened. I peered into Diane's sleeping face. She definitely wasn't dead; she actually looked pretty again. Her long black lashes curled up over her cheeks, giving her an angelic expression. I tiptoed downstairs and sat in the silence waiting for someone to get up.

CHAPTER 10

BY MAY, THE AIR, STILL DRENCHED from the moisture of April, had turned soft and fragrant. Winter finally slipped away, making room for drifts of violets that dotted the new grass in our backyard, marking the eighth month Robert and I were a couple. My finger, now elected as the place of honor for his ring, had developed a callus from the scotch tape wound tightly around the band so it would fit. For my birthday, Robert had given me a silver I.D. bracelet with my name engraved on a tiny oval that hung from its center. I never told him that he had spelled my name wrong, choosing a "y" instead of an "i" at the end.

That Saturday night was two weeks before the prom, and it was all I could think about. Robert picked me up on the pretense of a movie, but lately, most of our dates consisted of driving around Takoma Park and stopping at the Hot Shoppe to order hamburgers and milk shakes, and to check out who was there with whom.

Tonight was no different. We'd been driving around for an hour and Robert had done all the talking. I sort of wished he'd ask me about how I would feel when he left, or if I was going to be sad when he was not in school anymore, but he never asked about that. Lately he talked about getting into a fraternity and living on campus in a dorm the first year and all the stuff he was going to be doing, but none of it really included me. Sometimes I think he didn't really even know I was sitting beside him in the car because he always had so much to say about his plans, while I guessed I really didn't have any plans, except him. He was my only plan. I'd never honestly been sure why he picked me in the first place. The best I could come up with was that he thought I was funny. Like the other night when we were sitting on Julie's porch and I pretended to sing like Marilyn Monroe and made my voice real quivery, he laughed really hard at me and later told me I should try out for a school play. I'd never do that, but it made me feel good for him to say that to me. He said he loved me, but usually it was while we were making out, and he'd tried to slip his hand where it didn't belong. I guessed he liked me because I listened so hard to everything he said. I knew that I would have liked someone to listen to me that hard.

The night of the prom arrived and everything was set. Robert was coming at seven sharp. He knew the color of my dress but I didn't know what flowers he'd picked. That was a secret. I threw cold water on my face, brushed my hair back in a ponytail, threw on jeans and one of Daddy's old white shirts that hung almost to my knees. I didn't want to have to pull anything over my head and mess up my hair. Mom had already left to take Goldie to dancing school and open up the store, and Daddy was still asleep from his job last night.

Robert's parents were going to chaperone the dance; afterwards we were going to go to a party at Janice Kulaski's house and have breakfast at Nancy's. I was far too excited to eat the cereal Mom's left out for me, and instead gulped down a big glass of orange juice. Patsy was probably already at the corner waiting to walk to the beauty shop. This was her third prom and I relied heavily on her for leadership. I was more than a little nervous about the hairstyle I'd planned but decided to go for it.

The shop was filled with mostly senior girls I'd seen in the school halls but never spoken to. I didn't see another girl my age. Jackie DiMaggio was almost finished and everyone was gasping at how beautiful she looked. Her long brown hair was piled on top of her head and cascades of tiny curls fell down the back of her neck like Scarlett O'Hara. The lady fixing her hair was so fat the buttons around the middle of her dress kept coming undone and you could see the freckles on her stomach. Drops of perspiration formed on her forehead and she looked like she could do with a new hairstyle herself. She was holding a mirror so Jackie could see the back of her hair, but you could tell she was already thinking about the next girl standing beside her with a towel wrapped around her head.

Maybe it was the heat, but the smell of hair spray and the sound of the huge hair dryers all going at once started making me sick to my stomach. I wanted to run out of this place and forget the whole thing, but a young black girl had already handed me a ticket and pushed me into a chair to wash my hair. The water felt cool and with my eyes closed I actually began to feel better, but not for long. She wrapped my hair into a turban and told me to get into the chair right next to Jackie, who, to the annoyance of the fat lady, was taking her time at the mirror. Jackie was obviously taken by what she saw, until her eyes found me through the glass. I sort of smiled back but couldn't think of anything to say. I was even more shocked when she turned her chair around and looked directly at me.

"Robert tells me you're going to be at Janice's tonight after the dance." The smile had left her face but her voice was sweet as syrup. "I guess it must be pretty neat for you to be going to the

Good Girls Don't

senior prom. Robert told me you were real excited about it."

I still couldn't think of anything to say so I just nodded into the mirror like a dummy. My stomach had begun to really churn now.

"Well, I guess I'll see you tonight. Robert mentioned you'd probably be leaving the prom a little early," she gushed.

I sat stunned, watching her move through the beauty shop like she was riding on a float. Why had Robert told her all that stuff about tonight? He'd barely told me where we were going. I didn't know we were leaving early. Somehow the thought of him telling her how excited I was about the prom made me feel like a little kid. Not at all the way I wanted to feel today.

Jackie sure knew how to work a room, I thought. She was dressed in jeans and a white cotton shirt—not that different from what I was wearing, but on her it looked sexy. My stomach started making noises so loud I was afraid everyone in the shop could hear it, but by this time I was concentrating so hard on keeping down the orange juice I'd gulped down earlier, I couldn't think of anything else. It seemed to take forever for the fat lady to finish wrapping my hair into the little curlers that looked like chicken bones with rubber bands attached to the ends. By the time she finally stuffed cotton into my ears and wrapped the pink hair net around my head and shoved me under a dryer, I felt as though I was inside of a concrete mixer. There was no way I could keep the orange juice down. It took its own course—up and out. I tried to make it to the bathroom behind a curtain in the back of the shop but barely got to the center of the room, where I lost it on the linoleum floor. I stood staring at the disgusting mess of semi-digested orange juice mixed with long blonde stands of hair, and for a second I was so glad to have the sick feeling over I didn't even care. But after I realized how quiet everything was I couldn't believe what I'd done. Everything stood still except my head. I was mortified, especially in front of this holy audience. Somehow, the next thing I knew, I was sitting in a chair, although I couldn't recall how I got there. The black girl was putting a wet towel on my forehead and Patsy was beside me.

"Are you OK? Do you want me to call your mother? You look really white."

Unexpectedly, I began to think about how scared Diane had been the night of her abortion and how adeptly Mom had taken charge. C'mon, Patti, I thought, hold it together. All you've done is throw up. I bet every one of these little prom queens has done the same thing at some time in their prissy little lives.

"I'm fine now," I said, with a voice much louder than required. "I just can't smell that hair spray anymore. Sorry for the mess."

I look at the black girl who'd magically conjured a mop and bucket and was swishing away the orange yuck like it had never existed.

"No bother, honey, this place makes me want to barf sometimes, too," she said.

By the time the hair lady finished with me I looked as though I was wearing a sort of helmet decorated with tiny sausages randomly sticking out of the crown. When she gave me the mirror to look at the back of my head, half of the little sprayed sausage curls had already started to unravel, bobbing around my head like they were alive.

Mom was in the kitchen peeling potatoes when I got home. I brushed past her like I had something to do, completely ignoring the tangled mass of tortured curls jutting out of the top of my head. Mom had been against me going to the beauty shop from the start but I'd insisted, so after days of arguing, she'd finally relented. She couldn't understand why I wanted to look like everyone else, and laughed when I told her I wanted a bustle-back hairstyle.

She looked up before I could get out of her sight and I heard the sharp intake of her breath.

Good Girls Don't

"Jesus Christ, what did they do to you? You look like Medusa."

I was determined not to relive my whole miserable morning, but I couldn't hold back the tears any longer. I stood in the middle of the kitchen and sobbed out the whole story. Mom mercifully let me finish before she said anything.

"Well, I'm not going to say I told you so," she said, drying her hands on the dish- towel on the counter. "But, there is clearly no question that something has to be done about this hair. The sooner the better. Come over here and put your head in the sink."

I did as told, much too tired to argue. I hated that she was right about the beauty shop but I knew I couldn't possibly go to the prom like this. She didn't say much but scrubbed the gook out of my hair and wrapped it in a towel while she heated up a can of tomato soup. "Put tea bags on your eyes," she commanded. "It'll take away the red." I could never figure out how she knew this kind of stuff. She wasn't real big on hugs or telling me how great I was, but she was a good fixer. And she sure knew a lot of stuff. I had to give her that.

I can't believe how different I looked by the time Mom finished with me. She'd darkened my pale lashes with a sweep of sable brown mascara which made my blue eyes pop out like aquamarine marbles. I was surprised my eyes were so blue. It felt a little strange. It's not that I didn't like the person in the mirror; I just didn't know her.

Suddenly I didn't want to leave my room.

"I can't," I whispered to Mom. "I can't go. I don't look like me with this stuff on my face."

"Oh, yes, you're going," she said, tugging at the hem of my dress for the hundredth time. "You're going to walk into that dance and turn the corners of your mouth up. It's called a smile, and I guarantee you're going to hear a big wow from everyone at the dance."

"I don't want to hear anything like that."

"Oh yes, you do. After you've heard your first wow you spend the rest of your life chasing it around every corner. Here, take this purse I got for you. I put some Monopoly money into it. Now stand up straight. If you slump, you could lose that dress."

Scared and uneasy, I followed Mom down the stairs and into the back room where Daddy was reading the paper.

"You look…nice," he said, and then quickly retreated back to the paper—but I knew he was pleased because Daddy always got a funny smile on his face and made jokes when he didn't know what to say. I guess he couldn't think of a joke tonight and I was too nervous to fill up spaces, so I just let it be quiet between us.

It wasn't long before Robert knocked at the door.

My stomach clawed inside of me like it was holding a bag of birds. I'd been planning every detail of this night in my mind for over two months, and now that it was finally here I wanted to run upstairs and wash all the junk off my face. I didn't want to have to remember to stand up straight and keep this stupid dress up. I had no idea what I'd say to Robert's parents, and the thought of facing Jackie DiMaggio again today was more than I could bear. I glanced at Mom, who made an exaggerated thrust of her shoulders, her way of reminding me to stand up straight. I was afraid Robert was going to laugh when he saw me in this getup. I was beginning to feel as though I'd been caught playing dress-up in Mom's closet.

Robert walked into the living room smiling broadly, holding a shiny white corsage box. He looked all polished and scrubbed and I thought how lucky I was to have held on to him for eight months. He was wearing a white unbuttoned tuxedo jacket that draped casually from his broad shoulders, revealing a black cummerbund and pleated creamy shirt with little black studs for buttons. He wore the tuxedo like he'd been wearing one his whole life. I could barely look him in the eye. I took a big swallow inward and held it until I saw he was smiling at me. His smile was so big I began to relax a little.

"You look great, Patti," he said smoothly, not missing a beat. "No, you look beautiful."

I felt the blood rush into my face and remembered what Mom said about chasing the wows. I shrugged my shoulders, embarrassed. It didn't matter that lately he sounded like he was delivering lines from one of his plays. I smiled at him with open adoration I couldn't help. He opened the box and the scent of gardenias spilled into the room. I slipped the corsage around my wrist while Mom went into the kitchen to get the carnation in the refrigerator. Daddy had come downstairs just as we were leaving and said something about behaving ourselves. For just a moment, my parents stood next to each other, smiling and nodding, looking like anyone else's parents. They were looking at me like I'd just done something great.

Nothing prepared me for the spectacle of the hotel ballroom. Crystal chandeliers swayed from the highest ceilings I'd ever seen and alabaster columns turned the room into a palace from a fairy tale. I stood speechless in the center of a giant glass bubble that snowed confetti, afraid to blink because it might be a dream. Girls who I had grown used to seeing during the year in the hallways at school were transformed by swirling prom dresses of liquid rainbow, and the boys lost their awkwardness somewhere inside rented tuxedos. Everyone in the room seemed to have exceptionally good posture. It was almost like they were all auditioning for a school play.

I located a column in the corner of the room and made a beeline to lean against it until I caught my breath. But Robert had other plans and immediately led me onto the dance floor. I spotted his parents across the room sitting against the wall with the other parents who had volunteered to chaperone. I smiled at them until they smiled back. I guessed that meant I'd been approved. Actually they were lots easier than I thought they'd be. His father danced with me and told me "You're sure a pretty little thing." Robert's mother smiled a lot but barely spoke. She called me "dear" and complimented my dress, but never left her husband's side for a minute. The only remarkable thing about her was how furiously she tapped her feet to the music regardless of what the band played.

We danced close to each other to lush saxophone music and then gyrated and twisted to the new beats of the Lindy and the Texas Bop. We took off our shoes and danced in our socks and stockings until the soles were torn and shredded. And then some of us danced in our bare feet. We snuck off into dark corridors of the massive hotel and sipped Coca Colas laced with whiskey and smoked cigarettes until our throats were raw. I cheered as loudly as everyone else when Jackie was crowned prom queen and tried not to look too hard when Robert left me to dance with her. There were lots of trips to the crammed ladies' room, where girls pulled at crinolines and adjusted unfamiliar strapless bras in front of a full-length gilded mirror. A skinny black lady in a starched blue uniform and ruffled white apron sat on a stool collecting quarters from the girls who used her mirror.

When I returned to the ballroom Robert was huddled with a group of senior guys I didn't know. They were laughing in that way that boys laugh when girls aren't around. Robert hadn't yet seen me and I watched him throw back his head in big guffaws at something one of the boys said. His hand over his crotch as he grimaced in mock pain, which made the boys laugh even harder. I waited a few moments, pretending I hadn't seen all this, before approaching Robert and tugging on his hand to dance. His expression changed abruptly into an exaggerated look of rapt attention as he circled my waist with his arm, leading me away.

I enjoyed all of Robert's small attentions; he was such a pro at them. He never let me open a car door, always ran around to my side even when it was awkward. Once, he carried me up the steps to Julie's house because it was icy. I liked telling him when it was my time of the month and pretended to have cramps, even if I didn't. It made me feel close to him and helped me believe we would always be together. Like we were kind of already married. I'd begun scrawling Patti Marsden and Mrs. Robert Marsden all over my notebook and wanted to ask him if he wanted a girl or a boy first, but of course I didn't.

"Let's go out and find Dan and Julie," he said, his smile lasting a little too long. He'd taken his eyes away from me but the smile lingered, giving him a strange expression, like for a second he'd forgotten his lines. His eyes eagerly searched the room for something, all the while earnestly telling me how he'd never seen me look so pretty. He had a way of making his eyes real sparkly, as though he were about to burst with excitement over some surprise. I refused to pay attention to the frightening knot that was forming in my stomach. It began when I saw Jackie walking toward us. The light instantly disappeared from his eyes and color left his face, leaving him pale. He withdrew his hand from mine and jammed it into the pockets of his tuxedo.

"I told you so," he teased Jackie as she approached. "You didn't believe me but everyone knew you'd win."

"Oh, please," she giggled. "You were as surprised as I was and you know it. Don't pull your lines on me, Robert. You know I won't let you get away with that stuff. I know you too well."

I didn't dare touch him but desperately wanted to get his attention. I wanted him to stop looking at her and listening so hard to what she said. I began feeling unimportant, not an altogether unfamiliar feeling. Like sometimes at home when Mom and Daddy fought or when everyone watched Goldie at dance recitals.

I tried to keep my eyes averted, but I couldn't miss how soft her eyes became when she looked at him. I was too shy to feel jealous. If I were jealous I might have to compete, and she was far too removed from my world for that. But I could secretly hate her. She was talking so easily to him, like she didn't have to think before perfect words came out of her. I wished I could flirt with him like that. I was always so afraid I'd say the wrong thing.

I watched her glide into the center of another group who were waiting to pay their respects. By this time Robert had regained his composure and we were saying good night to his parents and heading for the door.

We found Julie and Dan jammed against the outside of their car, arms wrapped around each other, sharing a drink from a paper cup. When Dan saw Robert he didn't say a word but reached into the front seat and pulled out a paper bag, solemnly handing it to him.

When we climbed into our car Robert opened the glove compartment and pulled out a coke and two paper cups, which had obviously been planted earlier in the evening. He pulled the bottle of whisky from the bag, never asking me if I wanted it, and poured it into the coke. He handed me the cup as though it was something we always did. It never occurred to me not to drink it. By this time I was pretending so hard to not be me I'd forgotten who I was.

This time when he slipped his hand up to my stocking tops I didn't grab his hand; instead I thought, why shouldn't I let him? For the first time I allowed him to slide his hand all the way up between my legs. I finally forgot about Jackie or anything else for that matter. I closed my eyes tightly, sinking into darkness. God knows I'd been thinking so hard all day I was too tired for thoughts any more. His hand, like silk, massaged me at the same time he crooned into my ear. "You're so beautiful. Let me put it inside of you for just a minute."

I waited. Nothing awful was happening to me; lightning hadn't found its way into my heart and now I knew how much he loved me. I could tell by how tender his hand felt — gentle, almost polite. The liquor spread through my belly; his tongue filled my mouth and I began to move with the rhythm of his probing fingers. I knew a good girl would keep her legs tight together, but it was too difficult and they remained open, inviting. I knew I'd stop him soon — in just another minute. I must. That was when it happened. My head fell back and my body arched into his as though it were a rubber band being pulled by a force outside of me. The voice chattering inside my head, just moments before, became silent. It was the sound that startled me. Only seconds later did I realize the voice I heard was my own. I pushed Robert away with strength that almost toppled him on to the floor of the car. I began to cry, softly at first and then louder in big gasps.

"Oh God, Patti, I didn't mean to hurt you." He held me awkwardly and zipped up his tuxedo pants at the same time. "Are you OK? I didn't do anything. I promise. Please don't cry. Nothing happened. I'm so sorry," he said earnestly. "I wouldn't hurt you for anything."

When I straightened the stiff crinoline over my clenched knees I noticed a wet spot on the inside of my dress that was seeping onto my inner thigh. I instinctively drew my hand back and shivered despite the warm night. It felt like I'd put my hand inside a jellyfish. I didn't know what to say. I'd never seen Robert like this — so scared. His hands, clumsy, zipped up the top of my dress where just moments before he'd unzipped it. By this time I realized that both of my thighs were dripping wet and the stain on my beautiful green dress had come from Robert. It had all been so fast

I wasn't sure what had or hadn't happened. The only thing I was sure of was that I didn't want him to lose respect for me. I knew this was my fault. After all everyone knew that boys couldn't control themselves and weren't to blame. When Robert reached into his pocket for a cigarette I noticed his hand was trembling.

"I'm OK," I whispered, pressing my face into the silky lapel of his tuxedo jacket. "You didn't hurt me. It's just that I felt so much all at once. I'm sorry, I didn't mean to cry, please don't feel bad. You didn't do anything wrong." I pushed my face into his chest and wrapped my arms around him. "I love you, Robert," I said.

"I love you, too," he said automatically, the words perfectly spaced. I felt his back stiffen under my fingers as silence spilled over us.

The first orgasm of my life had taken me completely by surprise.

CHAPTER 11

I KNEW SOMETHING WAS WRONG WHEN ROBERT only called me once during the next three days. He sounded distant and preoccupied during our conversation — which lasted all of three minutes.

I spent the following days in a state of suspension. I sat on the edge of Daddy's bed and silently begged the phone to ring. I kept a biology book opened in my lap, pretending to study, but read not one word. Instead, I stared at the phone and made up desperate prayers.

"Please God, make him call. I don't care what he says, just let me hear his voice." I held my breath and counted to a hundred, promising myself he'd call before I passed out. He didn't call and I didn't pass out. Finally, one day after Mom had come home from work, she stood at the door, hands on her hips, leaning slightly forward — the pearl buttons on her shirtwaist pulled taut over her bosom — and stared at me. She released a sound like the beginning of a sigh. I continued to stare at my biology book as though she were not there, and looked off into space pretending I was memorizing plant parts. Eventually she left.

A small night table separated my parents' twin mahogany beds. Mom's copy of *The Good Earth* was wedged between a brimming ashtray and a glass lamp with Daddy's white shirt was flung over its top. Mom had covered the lamp to block out her reading light so Daddy could sleep. A pack of clarinet reeds had spilled on the top of the stained night table, but it was the small black phone in the midst of this marital clutter that was my object of obsession. I climbed into Daddy's unmade bed, strategically arranged schoolbooks around me in careful little piles so I could grab them quickly, and began my vigil. I noticed that dust had turned the numbers under the dial to gray and I tried to fit a corner of Daddy's sheet under the dial to rub out the grimy dirt, but all I did was fade the numbers more.

There was something deliciously decadent in this adolescent agony. The moments between possibility when the phone rang and the deep disappointment after I answered it became my drug. There was comfort in my job; it was clear and to the point. I must wait. No choice or confusion ---just wait. He had to call me. For God's sake, I had his ring. He couldn't pretend I didn't exist any-more. I slid underneath Daddy's covers where I escaped into a world so private I could create any scenario I chose. It was a place where I couldn't be diverted from my task and happy endings were always an option.

By Wednesday Mom had had about all she could take and I was forced to retreat into my own room, where there was no phone.

"Look at you, mooning every day over that boy," she explod-ed. "As if you can't find anything else to do. This is unhealthy — no, it's sick."

Ordinarily I closed my door, but on this night I purposely left it open slightly so there was no chance I'd miss the ring when it came. I had divided the house into zones where I could easily be the first to answer one of our two phones.

Finally his call came during dinner on Wednesday, exactly three days after the prom. I got the phone by the second ring and turned away from the dining room where Mom, Dad and Goldie sat eating. His voice was hurried but everything he said made perfect sense, as I knew it would.

His voice tumbled through the telephone line like he was out of breath. "Hi, sorry I haven't called but we've been practicing for graduation and I haven't had a second to think." The sound of his voice made me tingle and I almost laughed out loud with relief. I caressed the beloved phone, holding it close to my ear.

"Oh, that's OK. I've been busy too. I hardly noticed." I immediately wanted to swallow the words. They sounded stupid, like I'd been practicing.

"I mean, it's not like I didn't notice —"

"I'll pick you up after school tomorrow and we can take a ride," he interrupted, as thought I wasn't talking. "We need to talk."

I memorized each word of the conversation that night, scrutinizing every possible meaning. But he did call, I told myself, and everything is going to be fine.

The next afternoon, I stood in front of the gym holding my books in front of me like a shield. The day was humid, already thick with mosquitoes when Robert drove up in his green Chevy. I noticed the fixed smile on his face when he reached over and opened the door for me from his side.

"C'mon, get in, we'll drive over to the park so we can talk," he said a little loudly, like he was talking to someone with a hearing loss.

"Sure, the park's a good idea," I said, my hand instinctively reaching inside my cotton flowered blouse, grasping his ring.

Robert, suddenly shy, leaned against his door, careful not to touch me. I looked at his face, tight and unusually serious.

"Do you want to break up with me?" I hadn't expected to say this, but there it was like a splat breaking up the silence.

He pulled over onto the side of the entrance into the park and stopped the car.

After a moment, he said, "I do care for you, Patti, but it's time for us to move on. We're too young and I'm afraid you'll get hurt."

His response seemed far away, like an uninvited outside sound, seeping into the car. I watched him as though I was behind a one-way mirror. Briefly, a sense of calm overtook me, as though I was the one in charge, and then, just as quickly the calm turned to anger, a feeling to which I was unaccustomed and which I wore awkwardly. It was cold, clean adult anger and it was new to me. What he was saying didn't make sense. How could he not realize that this hurt was worse than anything else he could do? Had he lied when he said he loved me? Did he think I was cheap like the girls who go all the way?

"Why did you ask me to go steady with you in the first place?"

Robert looked at me. This question, it seemed, was not in the script.

"Don't you know?" he said softly. I shook my head, my eyes locked on his.

"It's because when I'm with you, you always make me feel good," he said, squeezing out words. "You look at me with those big eyes like I'm a big deal no matter what. And you're funny and sweet and you always act interested in everything I say. Nobody's ever really listened to me like you do. I know you really like me and I like you too, it's just that I'm going away to school and things are getting a little hot and heavy between us and I think you're getting too serious, and to tell the truth, you're just too young for me."

Good Girls Don't

I said nothing, but slipped the chain that held his class ring over my head and handed it to him.

We sat in the car that early summer afternoon at the end of an era, unaware of our fleeting innocence trying to say grown-up things and pretend that we knew about life. For me it was the first taste of raw heartache, and I'm pretty sure nothing had ever hurt more.

CHAPTER 12

IN THE TWO WEEKS FOLLOWING THE BREAK-UP I threw myself into my broken heart. When I tried to sing along with Nat King Cole on *They Tried To Tell Us We're Too Young*, I cried so hard my shoulders shook and the words came out in great heaving sobs.

The summer was a scorcher. Temperatures hovered in the 90s and the humidity was so thick I could almost see the moisture. It was the year most of our neighbors put air conditioners in their windows, but Mom had her own ideas, She found a window fan on sale at the hardware store and dragged it upstairs, jamming it into a window inside her bedroom. Then she left one window open downstairs to create a draft. She said that it would cool off the entire house. What it actually did was create a narrow stream of cool air barely the width of my shoulders. The only place in the house that was fit to sleep in was on the floor by the open window, which was where I spent most nights, at least when I wasn't on Patsy's front porch.

Patsy was busy getting ready to begin college, but she usually found time to listen to me. Together, we went through every moment of the prom and scrutinized details of precisely where his hands touched me that night and if I actually felt his penis or did

I just think I had. Hours were spent intensely debating whether I'd allowed him to go too far and would he or would he not lose respect for me. I assured my friend that my virtue was intact, as was my hymen, but each time I said this, another possibility was introduced as potential evidence. We even had a field trip back to my house very late one night to inspect the spot on the green dress, but since neither of us knew exactly what we were looking for it became a moot point. Since Patsy was older, she was expected to know more, but one night it occurred to me that I was the only one spilling my guts, and we got into a shouting match so loud it woke her father. When I realized she probably wasn't telling the whole truth about how far she went with boys, I ended my confessions.

It was Patsy who broke the news to me that Robert was dating Jackie DiMaggio again. We were lying next to each other on her front porch on top of sleeping bags during the steamiest night of the summer.

"I think she has his ring," she said, looking at me as though she might be expected, at any moment, to administer CPR. "I don't want you to find out from anyone else." She pulled out a Kleenex box hidden under the sleeping bag and handed me one before the news was completely out of her mouth.

Shocked and incredulous, I began rocking back and forth in a pose of grief that came far too easily these days. But the truth was I wasn't surprised. I had known this was going to happen the first time I saw Jackie in the beauty shop. There was almost a sense of relief in it being official now. I could go about the business of hating Jackie openly.

After this news my priorities changed. Although the mourning continued, it took on a militant, more pro-active direction. Most of my summer became devoted to the covert activities of spying, subterfuge and stalking. I entered into a world of late-night phone calls and drive-by stakeouts that occupied about as much time as the relationship had. If Robert and Jackie were seen together at the Hot Shoppe on a Friday night, by Saturday morning, I knew what she was wearing, what he was wearing, what they ate, and sometimes, even what they'd said to each other. I gathered a legion of spies recruited from girlfriends and girlfriends of girlfriends who called the house at all hours with reports of his whereabouts. I often called Robert's home phone number, only to hang up as soon as I heard his voice.

I knew exactly when Robert and Jackie broke up and every girl he dated after that. I knew when he joined the Sigma Nu Fraternity and I followed, with stealthy precision, the path of his fraternity pin, which landed on a new co-ed's bosom every couple of months.

Robert moved into college life with great ease and success, and although I was still in high school, I still found ways to document it all. I weaseled my way into fraternity parties and even dated some of his friends. Always on the lookout for new information, I chronicled cryptic messages into nightly diary entries. I became a skilled surveillance expert; only in retrospect did it occur to me that my behavior was reprehensible.

It took close to a year for my obsession to fade or at least dim. But finally, by my seventeenth birthday I'd filled out a little and although I still looked younger than my years, I was passably pretty. I was one of those lucky redheads that didn't have too many freckles and although my skin was fair, the sun turned it golden brown. My large eyes seemed to fit better on my face and a little mascara set off the blue to good effect. My red hair, which now fell well below my shoulders, was still my most obvious physical attribute and the one with which I was most easily identified. I grew used to wolf whistles from passing truck drivers and boys who hung from car windows shouting, "Hey, Red! Wanna ride?" or "Can you prove you're a real redhead?"

When Mom warned me not to trust boys — particularly ones

like Robert—any further than I could throw them, I'd dismiss the advice as Mom's usual distaste for things male. But for a while after Robert broke up with me, I began to see what she meant.

Ralph Provenzano proved to be the exception. One Friday night, early in November, Patsy was home from school for the weekend, and we spent the evening cruising Silver Spring together. We ended up later that night at the Tastee Diner ordering the usual bacon-and-egg late-night breakfast special when I first spotted Ralph. He was sitting across the aisle in a booth with a group of five or six boys all making rude fart sounds every time a girl entered the diner. It was impossible not to notice them. I glanced over to give them the most disdainful look I could muster. He was unsuccessfully trying to hide behind the menu, obviously embarrassed, when one of his companions picked up the saltshaker and began singing loudly into it, to the accompaniment of a chorus of shoobie-doobie-doos, that "all red-heads are cock-teasers with orange beavers." Ralph slid so far down into the corner of the booth he almost disappeared.

"Hey asshole, knock it off," he said to the guy singing, who paid no attention to him whatsoever. He looked so miserable it made me smile, even though his drunken friends, by this time, had gotten the attention of Hal, the manager, and it appeared a situation was brewing. Ralph shifted in his seat, flashed me a shy smile and threw his hands up in a gesture of apology. Hal walked over to their table and told them to pay up and get out. Everyone was used to this sort of thing happening on Saturday night, so nobody paid much attention—but when Ralph passed by me and stopped, I was surprised. His straight brown hair fell over his forehead, giving him a slightly disheveled look. He had a thin angular face, wore glasses, which he pushed nervously up on his nose, and was skinnier than he'd appeared sitting down. He was not especially good-looking, but there was something sort of sweet about the way he smiled. Not pushy but nice.

"Hey, sorry about my buddies. They've had a little too much to drink. They're not usually that rude, crude and unattractive," he said, leaning over the table. "Just rude and crude."

"I appreciated you trying to get those jerks to back off," I answered. "It was nice. Thanks."

"No problem. Well, see you around," he said, backing off. "Maybe I'll catch you here again."

"Do you go to school around here?"

"Yeah, I'm a freshman at Maryland U, but I'm from Patterson, New Jersey. We've just come from a fraternity rush party and I guess things just got out of hand. Sorry again."

Neither of us said anything for several seconds. He again moved to leave but suddenly changed his mind.

"You girls feel like company?" he asked. "I think I've about had it with those guys for tonight. I came in my own car. I doubt they'll even notice I'm gone."

"Sure," I said, a little too fast. "Have a seat." I figured he was interested in Patsy; most of the guys were. Patsy wasn't quite as enthusiastic.

"Do you live around here?" he said, looking directly at me.

"Yeah, " I stammered, "I've always lived here. I mean not always, but most of my life, since I was five years old. I guess that's practically all my life. I'm still in high school but can't wait to grad-uate." I'd have probably let him know the hospital where I was born if Patsy hadn't kicked me under the table.

"Yeah," he smiled. "I guess that counts for a lifetime. So what do you girls do on a Saturday night for fun?"

"Oh, mostly sit around in diners and wait for drunk college guys to be obnoxious."

He looked away, embarrassed, and I was immediately sorry

I'd said that. My head was racing to think of something clever to say but all I could come up with was, "What's it like in Patterson, New Jersey?"

"Not too different from here, I guess, except I don't know anybody here. And I know everyone there.

"I'd love to move somewhere I don't know anybody," I said, surprising myself.

"Yeah, I used to think that, too — but when you actually do it, it's not all that much fun. Gets kind of lonely."

"Well, the only place I want to go is home, " Patsy said, obviously bored with the conversation.

"If you don't live too far I can drop you off." Ralph said, looking directly at me,

"My mother would die if I got into a car with someone whose name I don't even know. What is your name?"

"My name? Ralph Provenzano."

"Provenzano," I repeated. "Italian, right?"

"Yup. Well, half."

"What's the other half?

"Jewish, my mother's Jewish. "

"Wow, me too," I said, swatting his arm, like we're related. "My mother's Jewish and my father's sort of Presbyterian except he never goes to church or anything. He's mostly just not Jewish, if you know what I mean. It's not like he has anything against being Jewish," I explained. "He just isn't."

"Yeah, I know what you mean. Except my parents never really got it together about what us kids were supposed to be. They're still deciding and I'm already 18."

We both laughed at the same time.

"By the way, my name's Patti, only I spell it with an "i.""

"Nothing very Jewish about Patti."

"I was supposed to have been born on St. Patrick's Day so

they named me Patti. But I was a week late."

By this time Patsy had her coat on and was poised to escape. I knew she probably thought this guy was a geek but I kind of liked him. He made me forget I was supposed to be cool.

"I guess you can drive me home," I said. "You don't look real dangerous."

"Are you sure?" Patsy said. "Don't let your mother know or she'll never let you go out with me again."

We sat there for a while not saying anything after she left. I surprised myself at how easy it was to just sit with him. I usually would have panicked with that much empty time, but the silence with Ralph felt OK.

"Do you have any brothers or sisters?" I said, finally.

"Yeah, nine."

"Nine," I repeated. "I've never known anyone with that many. I only have one little sister and that's enough. I always wanted a brother. Actually I had one but he died before I was born." For some reason I started telling him stuff I'd never told anyone. Not even Patsy.

We sat at the table for almost an hour. I told him about Robert and how crazy I'd gotten after we broke up and how I'd taken out my frustration by learning to type 100 words per minute. I couldn't believe all the stuff I talked about. He just listened and acted really interested, actually let me do most of the talking.

"I don't know why anyone would want to break up with you," he said. "You're the nicest girl I've met since I moved here. The girls at school all have their noses so high in the air it's a wonder they don't all have cricks in their necks."

We both laughed at that one until Hal told us we had to order something or leave. On the ride home Ralph showed me all the constellations in the sky. He said he liked Greek mythology

Good Girls Don't

and he'd teach me all about it if I wanted. I told him I did and wrote my phone number on the inside of a matchbook that was lying on the floor of the car.

It was after midnight by the time I got home. Daddy was working and Mom was stretched out in front of the TV snoring. The channel had signed off for the night and a test pattern was flashing on the screen, casting an odd shadow on her face. I woke her to go to bed and she didn't even ask me what time it was. I fell asleep thinking I'd talked more to Ralph Provenzano in one night than I'd talked to Robert in eight months.

For the next couple of months Ralph and I spent as much time together as possible. He lived on campus during the week but spent every weekend with me. It wasn't like I was in love with him, more like we were pals, but he was a guy, so it was different. He decided not to join a fraternity even though he'd been asked to pledge. He said he founds frats "too limiting." I loved when he said this. I knew that he was probably just shy but I didn't care. I'd never met a boy who talked like he did. I could tell he liked me but all he ever tried was a kiss goodnight and that was fine, too. I guess he knew I wasn't interested in anything more, even though we never talked about it. Ralph usually called on Wednesday or Thursday night to say he was going to be in the neighborhood on Friday and did I want to catch a movie or drive into D.C. with him. Usually we just drove around the Washington Monument or checked out Abe in the Lincoln Memorial, ate burgers in the car and talked.

It was Saturday, the last weekend before Christmas break, and we'd found a place to park at Haines Point on the Potomac River where we went to watch the planes land at the airport. Ralph was telling me a story about his Aunt Rosa, who was the family spinster. He walked in on her when he was thirteen, and she was doing it with the grocer who lived down the street. He said he was so embarrassed he tried to run away but instead tripped and knocked over a lamp and everybody acted like nothing had happened. He couldn't look at her for months.

We laughed so hard in that cold December night that puffs of our breath curled into the car and even that made us laugh even more. Ralph made all his stories about life in Patterson sound like they should be in a book or a movie where everyone was always laughing and eating spaghetti and cannoli around a big table. He said when he got home for Christmas his mother would make gefilte fish for Christmas Eve and his father would bring home codfish, and the kids had to eat both so nobody got their feelings hurt.

I told him about how Daddy dressed up the pheasant on our mantle piece and sniffed horseradish. He acted as though these were the most natural things in the world. The only thing I didn't tell him was how much I still thought about Robert. I knew that would hurt his feelings, and I liked him way too much to do that.

We sat for a long time watching the planes until Ralph broke the silence and asked, "what's the most exotic place you can think of?"

"Ireland," I answer immediately. "I've always had a thing about going to Ireland. Not sure why."

"Ireland," he said, surprised. "You kind of look Irish I guess, but I can think of lots more exotic places than that."

"I even like to say the word Irish," I confessed. "I like the way the air whistles through my teeth when I say it. Eye-rish. It's hard to say it and not smile." It was about that time that I noticed Ralph's arm was draped over my shoulder.

"I really like listening to you, Patti," he said. "I like you a lot." His glasses fell from his nose, as they often did, and even under his coat I felt his thin body tighten. He kissed me then. On the lips. A big, full-out kiss, not the usual peck like when we said goodnight. I kind of liked it; it was nice, even though it didn't feel anything like it did with Robert. I pulled away faster than I meant to, and I felt him sort of lose air as he moved back into the driver's seat. After a few silent moments, he started the engine.

We still hadn't said a word when we pulled up to the Tastee Diner. Fluorescent ceiling lights tinted the Friday night crowd as though in Technicolor. The jukebox blasted out the wrenching falsetto of the Platters singing full volume *Only You*. It felt like we'd just walked into the midst of a party going at full throttle. We took our seats, carefully avoiding looking at each other. I wanted to reach across the table and take Ralph's hand and tell him I wouldn't hurt his feelings for the world and let him know I actually liked the kiss, but the whole experience had made me crawl back inside of my shyness, so we both just sat staring at menus we knew by heart.

I glanced up from the menu just in time to see Robert walk in the door with some girl I'd never seen. I settled deep into the corner of the booth, trying my best to hide, but I was far too curious to stay there for long. A surge of excitement ran though me that I hadn't felt in a long time. A sound escaped my mouth. I cleared my throat to disguise it but Ralph noticed, even through the noise.

"What's the matter? Are you alright?" he asked. He reached over to pat my hand, studying it thoughtfully.

"You know, Patti, I really like you but I don't want to rush anything. Let's forget what just happened in the car. We'll go back to the way everything was. I don't want to upset you."

When I finally looked, I saw the sweetness gushing from him, but I was straining so hard to look over his shoulder at Robert that it was hard to act interested in anything Ralph said. Robert sat across from the girl, who didn't look at all like the type he usually went for. She never took her coat off, so it was hard to see her shape, but her face was wide and round, framed by short straight brown hair that she nervously kept running her hands through.

She talked nonstop and I wished like anything I could hear what they were saying. I could tell by the way Robert was sitting, all scrunched up, that whatever it was, it was not making him happy. He reached over and took her hand, and although I couldn't see his face, his back was toward me. It was definitely a consoling gesture, not affectionate.

I looked so hard over Ralph's shoulder that he finally turned around to see what I was looking at. It took him no time to get what was going on. I couldn't bear to look at his sad eyes, so I escaped into the ladies' room and waited there as long as I could, staring at my face in the mirror. When, finally, I found the courage to return, I walked directly in front of Robert. I smiled and looked right into his eyes and said, "Hi, nice to see ya", and right away I felt the old stab. It had been over a year since the break-up, but the pain of seeing him with another girl was like a fresh cut.

His face broke into a huge grin and he looked so genuinely glad to see me that for a minute I thought he was going to follow me back to my seat. He introduced me to the girl. Her name was Mitzi and she looked more than annoyed by my intrusion. I stopped at their table for just a minute, but by the time I returned to Ralph my head was so busy I could barely hear what he was saying. The encounter had left me incapable of continuing any pretense of conversation, and I desperately wanted to get out of there and go home where I could figure all this out. I couldn't help wishing Ralph would somehow disappear.

When I finally looked up to see Ralph, he was pushing his glasses so hard into his forehead I was afraid he was going to hurt himself. He stared at me dumbfounded.

"Do you always get so weird around that guy?" He blurted out. "If that's what all the noise is about, trust me, Patti, he ain't worth it. He's a big phony. Can't you see it? You're missing out on a lot by hanging on to someone who's so puffed up with himself

Good Girls Don't

he doesn't see anyone else. C'mon, let's get outta here. I want to go home. I don't like you very much this way."

I sat for a moment—speechless, shocked that Ralph would talk to me like that. I looked at him coldly before I grabbed my coat and practically ran to the car. I avoided any contact with Robert and his strange date. We drove home in frosty silence until we got to my house and I told him he had no right to say those things to me. I added that it would probably be a good idea if he didn't call me for a while. He didn't even walk me to the door, but before I left, he cupped my face in his hands and studied me thoughtfully.

"I don't know what to say to you," he said, hesitating. "It's time for you to get over him and move on. I hate watching you make a fool out of yourself over this guy."

His words stung but I brushed them off before I closed the front door. Ralph didn't know what Robert and I had been to one another. Nobody did. I knew that Robert really loved me and we would probably be getting married some day. I knew that as sure as I knew my name, address and phone number. And, I was even more convinced after tonight, the way he had looked at me in the diner. Nothing would ever make me think differently.

CHAPTER 13

MOM WAS ALREADY DOWNSTAIRS BY THE TIME I got up the following morning. I felt pretty crummy about Ralph and even considered calling him to clear the air, but truthfully, I was thinking more about Robert and his date.

I don't know how I got to the phone as quickly as I did on that Saturday morning. Mom, who was lost in a conversation with herself, was closer to the phone, but I was faster. I've often wondered how different my life might have been if Mom had been more agile that morning. Mom liked knowing everything that went on inside her house, and getting to the phone first was one way of doing this. There was no doubt that she would have hung up on Robert if she had ever heard his voice asking for me. She'd warned me about it enough times.

I knew within the first syllable who it was. The memory of that sound still causes my throat to catch. It crackled with certainty that we'd pick up exactly where we had left off, even if years had passed.

"Hi Patti, it's me. I know it's been a while, but I miss you today. Really miss you. Seeing you last night made me realize how much I need to talk to you." He flirted with his usual flair, but there was an unusual urgency to his voice.

Good Girls Don't

"You're right, it has been a long time. And, you're right again, you should miss me."

I surprised myself at how quick on my feet I'd become. I'd learned to hide behind glib one-liners, slipping in and out of a bravado I almost never felt. I felt the perspiration bubble up on my eyebrows and I was afraid I couldn't control my voice for much longer. I also knew Mom mustn't know was on the other end of the phone.

"Can you hold just a second?" I needed time to think. I took a big gulp of soda and forced myself to swallow very slowly while I watched Mom from the corner of my eye. She was spraying cleaner on the inside of the windows in the living room, apparently still lost in conversation with herself.

"Hi. I'm back," I said into the phone, sounding steady again.

"Can I see you tonight?" he said. "I've got some stuff I'd like to run by you."

"Sure, I guess so." By now I was practically whispering. "Pick me up in front of Patsy's house at eight."

I remained on the phone after he'd hung up, pretending I was talking to Ralph, using his name so often, that if Mom had been listening she'd have thought I was crazy.

"Who was that?" Mom asked half-heartedly, not really interested in the answer.

"Ralph," I answered easily. "We're going to a show tonight. Probably with Julie and Danny and some other kids. We might get pizza afterwards at the Villa Rosa in Silver Spring." I knew I was giving too much information, but I got lost somewhere in my own words.

"I'm going to meet him at Patsy's at eight so we can go to the late show, because he has to work until seven tonight at school. He always keeps so busy."

I knew I should shut up but the words kept coming, almost like it was someone else telling the story. Mom kept cleaning the windows and interrupted me in mid-sentence to tell me to finish the dishes in the sink. I was relieved to escape my own babbling.

I stood at the sink, my hands in hot soapy water, for a long time. I'd never won anything in a contest or gotten a prize or even been the best at anything, except maybe typing, but in that moment I felt completely redeemed. I'd won. Everyone I knew thought I was crazy, that he'd never come back to me. In their estimation, he certainly didn't love me. But I always knew differently, and after tonight we'd be a couple again forever. My hands were wrinkled and pink when I emerged from my thoughts. As I dried them, I convinced myself that Robert was going to ask me to run away and marry him tonight.

I hung up the dishtowel and started packing. I carefully laid two pairs of neatly folded white cotton panties, a pink rayon slip, my brown and white saddle shoes, socks, my best white angora sweater and a red plaid pleated skirt into my small overnight case and hid it behind the bush in the front yard. I figured if Robert wanted to leave right away I could grab the suitcase with little or no fuss and we could be on our way before Mom even knew I was gone. I knew Daddy would be playing a music job and not be home until late. I decided not to tell anyone, not even Patsy, that I was seeing him tonight. It would be a much better surprise that way. We'd tell everyone later. He might want to keep it a secret for a while and that would be OK too, but certainly not for too long. I felt the corners of my mouth pull upward and was surprised to see two spots of hot pink appear on my cheeks as I passed the mirror. My eyes were so bright they looked almost feverish. I spent the rest of the day in my room, watching the clock, minute by minute, until I could begin getting ready.

The night crackled with icy air as I ran down Baltimore Avenue to Patsy's house. As I turned onto her street, I saw her porch light was on, which meant she'd already gone for the evening. Probably had a date with one of her new college friends. I stopped in front of the huge oak tree in front of her house, careful to stay out of the light, and waited for Robert's green Chevy to turn down the street.

I waited about five minutes for his car to appear around the corner onto Albany Avenue, and for just a second I felt the sting of possibility that he might have forgotten or — worse — that he had been joking with me. My mind jumped around so quickly I couldn't keep up with it. Everything was upside-down. Of course he loved me. He looked so glad to see me in the diner — and hadn't he called the next day? Actually, he had called first thing in the morning. It'd be just like always. I felt his arms around me as soon as the headlights shined through the cold night. His car pulled silently up under the light, and as he reached across the front seat to open the door, I caught the reflection of his face in the streetlight. He was not wearing his usual smile but instead looked almost somber. It was the same expression I remembered from the diner the night before, with the girl. I'd never seen him like this. I jumped into the warm car and took a minute or so to stop shivering until I could finally speak.

"I hoped you didn't wait too long," he said. "I don't know why you wouldn't let me pick you up at your house, especially in this weather."

"I just thought it might be easier this way. You're not exactly the man of the hour in my house, you know."

He looked at me with a sad smile.

"I'm not anybody's man of the hour these days," he said, looking not at me, but out the window. He turned his head and I could see his eyes again. "Thanks for meeting me, Patti. I really needed someone to talk to, and you've always been such a good listener. Besides, I have something to tell you I don't want you to hear from anyone but me."

This wasn't going at all like I'd imagined. By this time I'd expected to be buried inside his arms, hearing his big laugh. I wanted to tell him about the suitcase hidden behind the bush and how happy I was to be near him again. I didn't even care that he wasn't saying the right words. I was sitting next to him in the car again and every cell in my body was focused on him. All I could think of was being touched. I held myself back from reaching over and touching the back of his neck like I used to when we drove together. But instead I sat with my hands in my lap, waiting. Finally he smiled and we relaxed a little.

"C'mon over next to me," he said, stretching his arm across the back of the car seat. "Let me warm you up. You're shivering."

I curled up under his arm, resting my head on his shoulder. Whatever he had to tell me couldn't take away this moment. I slipped my fingers inside his hand and we drove without speaking to Sligo Creek Park.

He parked the car in the same spot where we used to end all our evenings together. His body, warm and familiar, gave me the feeling of coming home. He kissed me with soft lips and everything slipped away.

"I've missed you," he whispered. "Everything always feels so right with you."

"I've missed you, too. I've never stopped missing you for a minute. I always knew you'd come back," I said, kissing him back, daring to slip my tongue into his mouth.

"I believe you've grown up a bit, Miss Patti," he teased. "I always knew there was potential—but who taught you to kiss like that? Don't tell me that guy I saw you with last night?"

"I get around, you know," I said, exaggerating my voice to sound sexy. He laughed, gently pushing me away, and looked into my face for a long time. It was hard to look at him for so long and not touch. He looked at me like it was the first time he really saw me. Something about his eyes frightened me. Maybe because it was the first time I'd really seen honesty in them, and I wasn't sure how to be with him this way. Or maybe I saw something that told me what would come next.

"You're growing into a beautiful young woman," he said, still staring at me. "I wish I were going to be around to watch you, because it'll sure be a sight to see. But something's happened and I'm afraid my life's taken a turn I didn't expect." He paused and took a deep breath. While he prepared to speak, I became aware of a strange feeling stealing over my body, like slow-moving paralysis.

"I've been seeing a girl for awhile, the one you saw me with at the diner. Her name's Mitzi Barton. She's in the University Theater Club with me and we were in a play together. It seems she's pregnant and it also seems I'm responsible. At least that's what they tell me. We're going to get married next week. As soon as this semester's over, in June, I'm getting a commission in the Air Force and I'll probably move to Texas with her. This isn't exactly the way I wanted my life to go but I have no choice. I'd be really stupid not to know how much you like me and I don't want to hurt you any more than I already have. I don't want to hurt anyone but it seems that's all I do. You're a wonderful, sweet, beautiful girl and you're going to find someone who will love you back as much as you know how to love."

His eyes never left my face and he was grasping my shoulders so hard they began to hurt. I'd been holding my breath and when finally it escaped, it left me feeling the most empty I'd ever been.

"Even when you left," I heard myself say, "and everyone told me differently, I didn't believe them. I knew you loved me." The words were out of place, but I succeeded in moving my mouth and uttering sounds. It was a feat.

"Oh, baby, I do love you," he said, and I saw tears in his eyes. "How could I not love you? You're the sweetest, purest thing that's ever happened to me. Timing has just never been on our side. You'll get over me, probably a lot faster than you think."

I flew back into his arms and kissed him harder than I knew I could. The only way I could tell him he was wrong was with my body. I turned my mind completely off, like I was shutting off the radio. It was too noisy. I had to touch him. Maybe if he knew how much I'd really loved him, all this would disappear. I slipped my hand underneath his shirt and touched his chest. He lay beside me in the car, his hand under my panties, opening me up. We didn't speak. Gently he pried open my clenched fist and placed it over his penis. I instinctively pulled away but he gently put it back and said, "Don't be frightened. It's just part of me." He steered himself directly over me and pushed against the moist gash of heat between my legs, pumping against me until I felt his body shudder and I pushed him away. It was over quickly, and he lay on top of me, his body melting over mine. Although he never penetrated me, he left my thighs soaked. My sobs were soon replaced by silence. We lay like this for a long time.

Good Girls Don't

CHAPTER 14

ROBERT WAS MARRIED SOMETIME during the following month. I never told anyone about that night with him. I felt pretty stupid unpacking the suitcase, and could think of no reason to share one more humiliation. Even though my insides felt like mashed potatoes, in a way there was a sense of relief — maybe even the beginning of something new. Robert was getting married and there was absolutely nothing I could do about it. Besides, it wasn't like he actually loved her or anything, so in a way nothing had changed too much. Not that it was easy to think of him climbing into bed with her each night — or, even worse, getting up in the morning with her. There was something so mysterious, so utterly married and grown-up about waking up beside someone each morning that it was hard for me to even picture it.

Christmas came and went quickly that year. I spent most of my time at Patsy's, only this time I made sure we talked mostly about her life, not mine. Daddy was busier than ever with music. Mom and I once again took our places in the back room. Just like usual I sat in the corner of the sofa in front of the fireplace, drinking hot tea and listening to Mom's stories. The latest was her version of Roberta's affair, and how she even let her boyfriend use her toothbrush. I thought Mom secretly wished for the courage to have her own affair, but of course, she'd never admit it. One night I got so comfortable, I just forgot. I told her I had run into Robert at the diner, and how he looked like he wanted to talk to me, but couldn't because he was with another girl. Mom, who sat with her feet curled up under her, in the big corduroy chair next to the fireplace, paused in mid-sentence and gouged her cigarette into the ashtray. I watched as the smoke coiled over our heads and floated out the open window. Her mouth moved as if she was still talking but no words came out. I then told her how close I'd felt to him that night, and even though he was getting married, I knew for sure he loved me. I really wanted her to know this. I didn't know why it was so important to me. Maybe if she knew he really loved me, she'd like him better. She spun around in her chair and said, "Don't mention that son-of-a-bitch's name in this house…ever."

Why did she hate him so much? I guessed it was like when Goldie fell out of the high chair and bumped her head and Mom threw the chair down the cellar. Hurting one of her daughters was not an option.

Ralph called me sometime in mid-January and we picked up pretty much where we had left off. The only difference this time was that I kissed him back at the end of our dates. We never talked about Robert. I guessed Ralph figured the kissing was my way of letting him know it was over.

About a month before my 18th birthday, on Valentine's Day, Ralph and I were leaving the Takoma Theater, where we'd just seen *Auntie Mame*. I loved going to the movies with Ralph. We talked endlessly about movie stars and stories, which usually opened up all kinds of other stuff to talk about. I was about to tell him how much I wanted to travel just like Auntie Mame, when he opened the car door for me and the smell of his cigarette hit me. My stomach began to churn so badly I had to ask him to stop smoking because I was sure I was going to throw up. We drove to the park and although it was February and freezing I stood outside, trying to breathe in air. I was so nauseous I insisted on going home.

The next morning I felt the sickest I'd ever been. Everything smelled like rancid butter. I made it to the bathroom in time to throw up, which was difficult, since there was nothing in my stomach and I was hungry. I wondered how I could be hungry and want to barf at the same time.

The next few days I threw up every morning, ate a huge breakfast, and by second period English class I was in the girls' room hanging over the toilet. By the end of the week I left school early, went home and opened all the windows in the house. I was sitting in the living room by an open window, still in my winter coat with a scarf wrapped around my neck. Mom came downstairs, shouting at me. "What in God's name are you doing? It's ten degrees in here." She touched my forehead. "Are you crazy?" she said, slamming windows shut all over the house.

"I don't know what's wrong with me. I feel sick. Everything smells bad. My throat aches. Maybe I have a brain tumor. I read in health class that people with brain tumors smell stuff."

"You do not have a brain tumor. Nobody's ever had a brain tumor in our family," she answered with her usual pragmatism. "You don't even have a fever."

Mom's hand was the only thermometer in the house. She could tell with uncanny precision, if we were sick enough to stay home from school. "Go upstairs and get into bed. I'll bring you some tea with honey. You probably have the flu."

When I came downstairs later for dinner and ate all the leftover spaghetti from everyone's plate, she surmised I probably didn't have the flu. By the middle of next week when nothing had changed, she said, under her breath, "If I didn't know better I'd think you were pregnant."

"Oh, right, Mom. Sure," I shot back, rolling my eyes.

"I've made an appointment for tomorrow with Dr. Cohen. Whatever's going on with you needs to be checked out."

I really didn't disagree with her but felt the need to complain half-heartedly anyway.

"I don't have a fever. I'm sure I just ate something wrong. I don't want to go to a doctor just because we have a smelly house."

Mom just gave me a look that meant the subject was closed. We didn't go to Dr. Cohen unless we had high fevers, earaches or strep throat. It almost always meant a penicillin shot and usually I'd do anything to get out of that. But this time, I was actually happy to see him if he could make me stop being sick.

I'd known Dr. Cohen for most of my life. He'd made lots of visits to our house when Daddy had pains in his legs and nobody knew why. He was there when Goldie and I had measles and even came to check on me when I got poison ivy so bad I had to stay in bed for a week.

"Make sure you tell him everything about when all this began," she said for the third time, while we were driving to the doctor's office. I nodded and agreed, but she was making a big deal for just a stomach-ache.

The receptionist called my name. Mom followed me.

"You don't have to come with me," I said. "I'm not a child. Wait outside. I'll know what to tell him. I'm the one throwing up, not you."

She paid no attention, as though she hadn't heard, and sailed right behind me. Dr. Cohen came out and gave her a big hug.

"Hi, Laura, you look much too healthy to be here," his deep voice boomed. He patted her on the back, never once looking at me.

"Hi, Sid, good too see you. Patti's been sick to her stomach. I want her checked out from head to toe. Apparently she thinks she's too old for me to be in here with her," her voice lowered like she was telling him an amusing secret, "but you know me, nervous Nellie. Just want to be sure everything's OK. You don't mind, do you?"

I never heard his answer because the nurse appeared with a cotton wrap in her hand and hurried me through another door and told me to take everything off. Everything.

I tried to hear what Mom was saying through the door but couldn't. I took off my clothes and wrapped the flimsy gown around me, not sure whether to tie it in the back or the front. I finally decided on the front and looked down at the stupid little pink flowers on it. I stood freezing in my bare feet when the nurse came back and told me to put on my socks and get on the examining table. Dr. Cohen walked in, followed by Mom. I refused to look at her. The doctor shoved a thermometer in my mouth and asked me to explain if I was sick all the time or just now and then.

I pointed to the thermometer in my mouth. Smiling at me for the first time, he told me to just relax for a minute.

"I think it might be a good idea to give Patti an internal examination. She's never had one and this is probably as good a time as any," he said, still looking at Mom.

"I thought you might want to do that, Sidney," Mom answered. "Which is exactly why I thought it might be a good idea for me to be here. It'll make Patti feel more comfortable."

He slid the thermometer out from my lips. "When was your last menstrual period?" he asked, looking at the thermometer.

"I don't remember," I said. I really didn't. I tried to, but I was so taken off guard I couldn't think straight.

"Patti, is there any reason to believe you could be pregnant?" he asked quietly. "Have you had sexual intercourse in the last few months?"

Mom was still standing in back of me. I couldn't see her but I could feel her. Blood rushed to my face and I felt heat press through my body. Why was he asking me this?

My mind raced back to the last time with Robert. I knew we hadn't done it. Not really. He pushed against me but that's not what the doctor was talking about. The room was so quiet I could hear the doctor's stomach grumble. I wanted to turn around to see if Mom heard too, so we could laugh about it on the way home. I tried to concentrate on his questions. He was the doctor and could ask me anything he wanted. And I had to answer. I sat there with my feet hanging down from the cold table, wearing only white bobby socks and the flowered gown and, against my will, I told them about making out with Robert in the car. Then I had to tell them that he was married. And, I even had to tell him how my panties were off when he pushed up against me. When I said that, Mom let out a terrible sound. I thought I was going to be sick all over the table but his questions kept coming.

"Did he ejaculate inside of you?"

"I don't think so."

"Did you feel him enter you?"

"No. I mean, not really."

Did you notice any blood after the event?"

"No."

"Was he lying on top of you?"

"Not exactly."

"Was it the first time you ever had intercourse?"

"Yes. I mean, no. I've never even had intercourse."

"Please try and speak up, I can't hear you."

"I'm sure I can't be pregnant," I whispered. "I'm still a virgin. I've never had intercourse. There was never an event."

I could barely say words like "intercourse" and "ejaculation." They sounded horrible. Like in health class when all the guys giggled about the human reproduction part and they showed that weird movie. I hated those words. That's nothing like what Robert and I had done.

Good Girls Don't

"Well, let's just take a look here and see what's going on," Dr. Cohen said. "I'm going to be very gentle, Patti, and use the smallest instrument I have, so I don't want you to be frightened. I'm going to tell you everything I'm going to do before I do it so you'll know what to expect. And it's perfectly OK if you want Mom here. She can stay right where she is."

"It's alright Mom. You don't have to stay." I desperately wanted her to leave. Why didn't she just leave?

"I'll be right here," she said, grabbing my hand. The doctor had some kind of lever at the end of the table. Then I saw these little stirrups on either side. He placed my feet inside the straps. I squeezed my eyes shut to escape. When I opened them I looked hard at my white socks raised up. There was a tiny hole in the heel; I didn't look at Mom standing beside me. Dr. Cohen pushed that cold thing up inside of me. It hurt. I want Mom to let go of my hand: leave, go away. He took a long time and when he was finally through he told me to get dressed and meet him in his office.

"We won't say anything to Daddy about this. He's not a strong man. He won't be able to help," Mom said to me, her voice calm and measured.

"Mom, I didn't do anything wrong."

"The first wrong thing you did was bring that boy home. Didn't he ever hear of rubbers? And you, for Chrissake, do you even know when something's inside of you? Now get your clothes on and let's hear what other great news Sydney has for us."

In the bathroom, after I got dressed, I heaved into the toilet bowl, and then sat down on the toilet. None of this made sense. It was all a big mistake and I was sure when we got into his office he'd clear it up. He probably had to ask girls those questions if they'd never had an internal examination.

Dr. Cohen was seated behind a large mahogany desk covered with glass. The only thing on it was a fancy gold pen set, a round glass paper weight he kept picking up and putting down, and a silver framed photograph of a lady with black hair pulled up on her head in an old-fashioned upsweep. Her arms were wrapped around two small boys looking very serious, one wearing rimless glasses too big for him. I looked at the diplomas from Pennsylvania State University and George Washington Medical School on his wall. I took the chair next to Mom, across from his desk.

"I can't tell anything conclusively until after the rabbit test, but you're displaying symptoms of pregnancy." He cleared his throat and continued looking at Mom. I waited for the part where he told me that it was impossible, but he didn't. "Also, there is an irregularity on your left ovary which may be causing you discomfort. It appears as though you have a cyst on it, almost the size of a grapefruit. It must be removed, which will require surgery. I think the operation should be done by a gynecologist."

He pulled a small tablet from his pocket and began writing something on it. "This is the name of a doctor at Doctor's Hospital downtown who I think you should see. In the meantime, leave a urine specimen before you go…for the rabbit test."

The room began to spin. I felt like someone had just turned up the volume in my head, it was screaming so loudly. The silver-framed photograph looked out of focus. Tears hung in my throat and my voice came out louder than I meant for it to.

"I haven't done anything wrong. I didn't do it. We didn't do it. I didn't go all the way. I stopped before it happened."

I was sobbing and felt like I was going to throw up again. Dr. Cohen told me to calm down, that we didn't know anything for certain yet. He told Mom to take me home and put me to bed and not to "hang the crepe on the front door yet."

Mom and I said nothing in the cab on the ride home. Thick silence, like stale air, hung between us.

Goldie and Daddy were eating leftover meatloaf in the

kitchen when we arrived home. I could hear Lucy and Desi on the television in the back room. Mom nodded permission for me to escape upstairs. I heard Lucy and Ethel shrieking with laughter as I climbed the steps to my bedroom. I fell on top of the bed and tried to remember what I was doing during my last period. My eyes burned with tears as I fell asleep counting weeks on my fingers. I didn't wake up until late the next day.

Dr. Cohen came to our house a day later. Mom answered on the first knock. I saw them from the top of the stairs. It was the first time I'd seen him without his white coat. He wasn't even carrying his black doctor case. He followed Mom into the back room, sat on a dining room chair she'd pulled to the edge of the room. Mom was in the corduroy chair and I sat very straight on the couch. My back didn't touch anything.

"I ordered two rabbit tests because I wanted to be absolutely certain," he said. He made an elaborate gesture of reaching into his pocket and slowly pulled out a neatly folded handkerchief. As in slow motion he began to clean his glasses.

"Patti is definitely pregnant." His words dropped into the room, heavy and hard. He spoke only to Mom, as if I were an innocent bystander listening in on a private conversation. "If it's any consolation, it's a textbook case. I really didn't believe the first test. I thought it must be a mistake so I ordered the second one. I've never seen anything quite like it. Whoever that kid is, he's got Olympian sperm."

I didn't hear much after that. His words were out of tune, like a screechy violin. Maybe they were talking about someone else. I tore my eyes from the window, where I had been staring at a bird perched high above in a tree, and looked at Mom. Her face was all crumpled. She sank back into the big chair, worn and tired, and said nothing.

"The first thing that has to be addressed is the cyst," the doctor continued. "Make that appointment with the gynecologist as soon as possible. Laura, between you and me," he leaned forward, "there's a good chance she'll abort if the surgery is done quickly. All that guy needs to do is just nudge a little in the right place. You never know if he will or not, but it's a possibility."

"I've already set that up," Mom said tersely. "We go the day after tomorrow."

"Good!" He shifted his gaze onto me for the first time. "And as for you, young lady, just do everything your mother says to do. She's a strong woman and I have no doubt she'll make the right decisions. I don't know why you kids think you have to rush everything." He shook his head slightly. "You'll get everything in, you know. Just take your time."

I tried to speak but a wail, loud and high pitched came out of my mouth. I felt my head spinning out of control as I jumped off of the couch. There were no tears, just dry sobs. "No, your rabbits are wrong," I screamed. "They're wrong! Why won't you listen to me? I didn't do it. I'm a good girl. I can't be pregnant. I can't."

Mom put her hand to her forehead, as though for support. She leapt out of the chair toward me, but I was faster. I reached the front door, pulled it open, and there was Goldie on the front porch coming home from school. She and her friend, Anne Marie, were singing *Mairzey Doats* and giggling so hard they were holding each other up for support. I ran past them, almost knocking Anne Marie down. Mom stopped at the open door, the doctor beside her, and they all watched me run down our street.

I came to the creek and found the tangled root that jutted from the bank. I nestled into it, letting it cradle me like I'd done since I was little. I sat for a long time in the chilly afternoon. Nothing made sense but the creek, the tangled root, and the cool air. I made a bargain with God that if I didn't cry or make any

Good Girls Don't

sounds it meant this was all a dream. I'd come here to cry but instead I slept. I didn't hear Mom when she found me.

The next few weeks were like no others before. There were days when I noticed everything, like the overly polite way Mom spoke to Daddy, who still knew nothing, and other days when I was numb and everything was a blur. On those days I stayed in bed late and ate Saltine crackers that Mom had laid out for me. She said if I ate them as soon as I woke up, I wouldn't be so sick. She also put lemon drops in bowls all over the house. She said they helped when she was pregnant. I took all my directions from Mom, who had a new plan every day. She never lectured me. She actually didn't talk much to me, but mostly to Roberta and Ninny. I got most of my information from listening to her phone conversations while hiding at the top of the stairs.

Two days before I was scheduled to go into the hospital for the grapefruit operation, I heard Mom tell Roberta that she'd found someone if things didn't go well. She said that Mrs. Gregory, a friend from the dancing school, had a brother who was a doctor, and he had found a way to help someone she knew last year. Apparently Mrs. Gregory's brother wasn't the helpful one, but he'd make a call to someone he knew in Baltimore, if necessary. I'd never even been to Baltimore. Although it was just an hour away, it seemed like another country to me. The only thing I knew about Baltimore was that the guys in school joked about sneaking off to go there for strip shows.

After Mom hung up the phone I laid there thinking how much I wished I could call Robert and tell him everything. I pretended that he would march into our house, straight into my bedroom, and announce to everyone that he loved me and we were getting married, and nobody could stop us. He would put his arms around me and lead me out of the house and into his green Chevy. We wouldn't even look back. I was so lost in my dream I didn't hear Mom come into my room.

"Daddy's home," she announced, her voice never wavering. "I told him." It was the first time I saw tears in her eyes. "He's in the bedroom. Go to him."

"I can't," I said. "Don't make me see him. Please! Why did you tell him? We can go to Baltimore. He'll never know."

"Nobody said anything about Baltimore," she answered, her voice rising to a dangerous pitch. "I can't take too much more, Patti. Go in there and talk to him. Now!"

I opened the door to their bedroom and saw Daddy standing in front of the closet. His freshly pressed tuxedo shirt hung over his boxer shorts and his long black socks were pulled up almost to his knees. His bow tie hung undone around his neck. His hands seemed oddly out of place, dangling in clumps from his unbuttoned cuffs. I could barely raise my head to look at him. His face was ragged and smeared with tears.

"Daddy, I'm so sorry—I'm so sorry," I whispered. I knew I was going to cry, but what I really wanted was to die. I walked toward him and tried to put my arms around him, but Daddy was unaccustomed to hugging, and I was equally uncomfortable feeling his hugs. So we stood awkwardly together, each waiting for the other to speak. When finally, he broke the silence, his voice was strangled.

"That bastard prick did this to you?"

I'd never seen Daddy cry. I couldn't look. We stood together for a long time, but said nothing. Then the door opened and Mom's footsteps came into the room and stopped. I felt rather than saw her sit down on the edge of the bed, in back of me. Daddy walked to the window sobbing uncontrollably. I followed him, trembling all over, and touched his hand.

"That son-of-a-bitch prick," Daddy kept saying over and over to no one in particular.

Mom broke in. "There's no time for that. There are decisions

Good Girls Don't

that have to be made—and I hate being the only one that makes them." This time there was hot anger in her voice.

My throat was tight. I couldn't help the sobs.

I spent the next few days in bed, until it was time for me to go to the hospital. I listened to the sounds of our house—dinner, the phone ringing, the front door opening and closing. I cracked my door late at night, after I was sure Goldie was asleep and Daddy was home from a music job, so I could hear Mom and Daddy argue about what was going to happen to me. I felt like an ink blotter. I absorbed their thoughts and ideas and even their pain, but never spoke of it to anyone. When Mom came to tell me that Patsy was on the phone or Ralph wanted to talk to me, I pretended I was asleep. Mom brought my dinner up on a tray as though I had the flu or cramps.

I stayed like this until the evening Uncle Charlie picked up Mom and me up to go to the hospital. Daddy had to work that night, which was what he did almost every night lately. I guessed everyone was hoping that when they took out the grapefruit, the baby would just go away, too. I knew I did. I wanted so badly for this to happen that I didn't even feel scared about the operation. Uncle Charlie leaned over and told Mom that everything would probably be fine afterwards, and just to "hold on." Mom, who was talking non-stop, told Uncle Charlie she'd just take it one step at a time, but right now she just wanted to get this part behind her. I could tell she was nervous because she always acted mad when she was scared. She turned around and looked at me really hard in the back seat and said, "I've hired nurses around the clock to take care of you after the surgery. I'm a complete wreck, but at least I'll know you're getting the best care possible. Maybe then I can get at least one night's sleep." Then she shook her head back and forth and said to herself, "How did I get such *tsuris*? One minute you think everything's fine, your kid's OK, and the next thing you're taking a ride to the hospital. You know I'm really not as strong as everyone thinks I am." I said nothing, but wished Uncle Charlie would drive faster.

News of my surgery spread quickly among my friends. All anyone knew was that I was having a "female" operation, but apparently this information exalted my stature into a mysterious realm; one requiring somber respect. By the time I'd settled into my room to wait for next morning's early appointment with the surgeon, I'd begun to feel better. My room started to fill up with kids. Patsy and her mom were the first to arrive, bringing a gift all wrapped up like a birthday present. Patsy and I, who talked to each other every day, acted as though we've just met — like we'd forgotten that up until now we'd known everything there was to know about each other.

Next, Ralph came in, poking his glasses as usual. He was so nervous he just sat in the corner and stared at me, wearing a worried expression. All the while Mom sat in a chair by the window, watching.

A nurse came in to tell everyone it was time to leave, but no sooner than she had got it out of her mouth, the door opened, and Robert walked in. It was as though all the air left the room as he walked right to my bed, picked up my hand and said, "I just heard about all this tonight. Why didn't you call me?"

I didn't answer, but looked at Mom, who by now was standing. Her lips were pushed so tightly together they appeared to be lost somewhere inside her mouth. The only sound in the room was her loud breathing. She looked away, but not soon enough. No one in the room had missed that look. Her eyes turned so fiercely black I was sure they would wilt all the flowers. It took less than the blink of an eye for the room to evacuate, except for me, Mom, and Robert.

Mom stood up, squarely facing Robert, every word carefully

Good Girls Don't

controlled as though she'd been rehearsing this for a long time.

"I don't know how you could possibly have the nerve to walk in here like nothing has happened. My daughter is about to undergo serious surgery tomorrow morning and I don't want to cause her any more pain. You have ruined her life, but I will grant you five minutes, because I will not upset her by a scene. My husband will be here soon and I strongly suggest you're out of here by the time he gets here."

Robert looked bewildered. "I don't want to cause anybody any pain," he said, "especially Patti. I just heard she had to have an operation and I want to wish her good luck. I'm sorry if I did something wrong." His voice was now trembling. "I think the world of Patti."

Mom walked out into the hall, leaving the door wide open. Robert glanced at the door but made no move to close it. He pulled up a chair by the bed and put his hands out in a gesture of confusion.

"What was that all about? Is she mad because we broke up? I always thought she liked me. What the hell's going on?"

"I'm pregnant." I said, unable to get the words out fast enough. I'd practiced telling him so many times; the words tumbled out in chunks, like a tsunami crashing into the room. "That night in the car—I guess we went further than I thought—and, I have a grapefruit on my ovary—I mean not a real grapefruit, but everyone seems to be worried about it—and I'm sick all the time and all I ever wanted to do was get married to you—but you're already married—maybe Mom will take me to Baltimore to Mrs. Gregory's friend to get an abortion—or maybe I'll go to Pittsburgh and hide out with her family and have it there—maybe Mom will adopt it or I'll give it to someone who really wants it who can't have kids—Mom thinks of something new every day and I don't know what to do—so I just do whatever she says—all I really want is for it to go away, but I know it won't—I wanted to call you so bad but I was afraid because you're married and I know it wasn't really your fault—it wasn't anybody's fault—even though Daddy called you a prick and cried and Mom wanted to know why you didn't use a rubber."

Robert squeezed his eyes together like someone who's trying to dodge the first blow but knows he can't. Words kept sneaking out of me in choked syllables and half-stuffed moans. Tears spilled down my face and smeared into the snot dripping from my nose. I tugged at my new silk bed jacket and rubbed my nose in it. I waited for him to tell me he would immediately divorce Mitzi and marry me and we'd have our baby and find an apartment and we'd wait to have a big wedding after the baby was born. This is what I wanted to hear.

Instead, he dabbed at my eyes with the sheet and said nothing. His mouth was open like he was about to speak, but nothing came out. He just stared at me like he was waiting for more. Only there was no more, so he looked away and we both stared at the blank wall.

When finally he spoke, his voice was so quiet I barely heard him. "Not you, Patti. This can't be happening to you, of all people."

I wanted to say he'd gotten it wrong. That it was happening to us, not just me, but I didn't have the courage. Actually, I was so happy to have him here, even for a moment, I didn't say anything. Maybe he was right. It was happening to me. He was going to leave in a few minutes and I'd still be here, with the baby inside of me, not him.

"What can I do?" he said. "I'll do anything. Just tell me."

Mom walked into the room in time to hear this and answered for me. "I'll tell you what you should have done. You should have thought to put on a rubber. And, I'll tell you what you're going to do." Her voice rose to a shout. "You're going to get the hell out of here and never show your face around my family again. You've already done more than enough." By this time she was yelling so loud that a group of nurses had stopped outside the door. With an effort, she lowered her voice. "Rest assured, I do not hold you entirely responsible. My daughter is well aware of the facts of life and allowed this sordid thing to take place. Unfortunately, she does not know how to separate sex from love. She does not know that when a man truly loves a woman he also respects her and these two go hand in hand, and not one without the other. A man who loves a woman does not place her in a precarious position. We don't need you; we never will. I want you to know something."

She paused, dropping her voice to a whisper. Even the nurses standing at the door didn't dare interrupt. "I am Patti's mother and I'll protect her like an animal. You have taken away her most treasured possession: her reputation. I have to also consider my younger daughter, whose reputation could be at stake because of this, not to mention an unborn child who will live with the stigma of being born out of wedlock. Then, my husband, who is well respected in the community, where, I might add, we have lived for over 20 years. You want to know what you can do? Never come near any of us again."

"Yes, ma'am," Robert muttered, staring into the floor. Although he was almost a foot taller than Mom, by the time she'd finished, he had withered, and actually appeared smaller than she. "I'm so sorry, Mrs. Hawn, I feel awful. I wish there was something I could do."

He looked so grateful when the nurse came in and told him he had to leave that he didn't even glance back as he left the room. The nurse gave me a shot of something, and when I awoke I had the worst bellyache I'd ever had. The grapefruit was gone, along with my ovary. But the baby was still there.

By April, although I'd completely recovered from the surgery, the hope that I'd miscarry had vanished, replaced by a new plan. Since everyone thought I was still getting over the operation, it was easy to avoid my friends. I didn't return to school, instead spending long hours alone in my room.

Late one night Mom came into my room and perched on the edge of my bed. I knew she had something to say, probably another plan. She looked like she was going to cry and for the first time I noticed dark circles under her eyes. Her short curly hair looked unwashed and lifeless.

"I made a call to Mrs. Gregory's friend," Mom began. "The one who knows the doctor in Baltimore."

I listened more intently when I heard the word Baltimore.

"He called me back today and said he'd meet us there and maybe he could help. Actually he said he could help. I don't know, though; it seems so risky."

I nodded in agreement, but Mom didn't notice. She'd stopped looking at me and instead was looking over my head, like there was someone in the back of the room she was talking to.

"What if something goes wrong? I don't know… I just don't know…Roberta thinks I should do it, but Ninny feels you should just go to Lizzy's in Pittsburgh and have it. Lizzy's pregnant and I know she'd take you in. I told your father we could adopt it but then, of course, everyone would know."

I nodded again. " I'm not sure I can take you to Baltimore. I'm just not sure I can do that."

Mom, by now, was having a complete conversation with herself, and I was once again taking that familiar walk, eavesdropping through her head. For a moment I wondered what I'd say if she asked me what I wanted to do.

I thought it would be scary to have an abortion, but it would also be scary to go to Pittsburgh and live with Mom's cousin. It would be really scary to have a baby and give it to Mom to raise.

What would the baby be? My little sister or brother? Or maybe I could just move somewhere far away and never see any of them again. Maybe I could move to New York and lose myself in a big city, and live in an apartment by myself and keep the baby. Or Mom could send me money. Or I'd get a job typing. I guessed it would be better to go to Baltimore even if I died.

It was a muggy, heavy evening—cloudy, with the promise of rain, typical of April in Maryland. I sat in the back seat of Uncle Charlie's new Kaiser/Fraser, looking at Mom and Uncle Charlie in the rear-view mirror. The lights from the highway flashed into the car every minute or so, lighting us up. Uncle Charlie's cigar was making me sick, but I didn't tell him. I huddled into the corner and pressed my nose into the back seat and the smell of his new car. Somehow Uncle Charlie's cigars never smelled that bad. It got all mixed up with his other smells, like pipe tobacco and the spearmint Chiclets that he was always popping into his mouth. Uncle Charlie's fedora was plopped square in the middle of his head, and he was hunched over the seat of the car, looking from the back like a huge stuffed brown bear. Uncle Charlie was always behind the steering wheel of a car. He was the official driver for our family. I remembered the time when we were driving on the Pennsylvania turnpike returning from our annual visit to Mom's family, when Goldie got into Ninny's purse and Mom thought she had eaten her thyroid pills. She made Goldie drink coffee at every Howard Johnson for five hours. When Goldie threw up all over Mom's green suit, and I did the same from the other side, Uncle Charlie, never said a word, just kept driving until we were home, even though the smell never really left his car. He was the only one in the family who bought a new car ever year. Said he had to do it to look good when he called on customers to sell them the diaper service, or the paper products, or whatever he happened to be selling that year.

I looked at the back of his head and noticed his thick gray hair curling around the back of his worn felt fedora. I wished I were back on his front porch putting curlers in his head and playing beauty shop with him again. Uncle Charlie always let us kids do anything to him. When I asked him how he got his glass eye, he said he got beat up by hoodlums in Brooklyn who hated little Jewish boys with big mouths.

Mom read directions to Uncle Charlie from a piece of paper she pulled out of her purse. Streetlights shone on blocks of small boxy houses with clean white stoops, all lined up in neat rows, like an empty crossword puzzle. We were supposed to meet Mrs. Gregory's friend at the corner of one of these streets, and he was going to drive us to the doctor's house. Mom had told me the details so many times it almost seemed like a movie I'd already seen. The man who would do this was a real doctor who lost his license. He couldn't practice medicine anymore, but Mom said it wasn't his fault, that he'd been railroaded by his ex-wife, who was out to get him. He was really a nice man who used to be a doctor, just like Dr. Cohen, only now he did these abortions to help girls who got in trouble. I guess that would be me. I was for sure one of those girls in trouble.

Curled into the corner of the car, I thought of the baby inside of me. Up until this very minute, this baby had been no different to me than the grapefruit that the doctor took out. All I wanted to do was get it out of me. It was taking up my whole life — had changed everything. Mom said it had ruined my life. But that couldn't be true, could it? After all, I'd never even really done it with a boy, so how could my life be ruined already? It was hard to think of me as a mother. Mom was a mother. I was a daughter. I placed my hands over my flat tummy and tried to imagine a tiny pink baby floating around inside of me. The image disappeared as quickly as it came. I pulled my hands away and tucked them out of sight, under my thighs.

Uncle Charlie glided the car through the dark Baltimore neighborhoods, slowing down to peer out at the street names. We stopped at an intersection to allow a hollow-faced old man to cross the street. When he passed under the streetlight, his face looked dry and yellow, and he stared into our car like he was asking what business we had on his street. I couldn't help wondering the same thing. We passed a stretch of cheap apartment buildings behind chain link fences, a liquor store, a Chinese restaurant and a boarded up grocery store with "Jesus Saves" childishly scrawled across its windows.

Mom had stopped giving directions to Uncle Charlie and was staring out the window. She pressed down the button that locked the car door and told me to do the same. Uncle Charlie gave her a sideways look, as though to ask for the next landmark, but she said nothing, just pushed her purse further into her lap and stared straight ahead. Fear began to jab and prod me, and I felt as though a large basketball was lodged in my stomach. I waited for Mom to say something. Anything. When finally I couldn't stand the silence I asked, "Are we almost there?" It's the first time I'd spoken during the entire journey and my voice sounded hoarse.

She snapped back at me "to just hold tight, we'll be there shortly." She jerked her head around and looked at me huddled into the corner of the car. She let her hand fall over the back seat, where it grazed my knee. Her touch, like an electric current, reminded me that Mom would never let anything bad happen to me.

"Laura, for crying out loud, read the directions to me," Uncle Charlie said. "I thought you said you knew where the hell we were going. I'm not letting either one of you out of this car around here.

I don't care who this guy is or how good he is."

The words were no sooner out of his mouth than Mom hissed at him to turn the car around and drive us home.

"Let's get the hell out of here. I must have been completely insane to bring her here." She spilled out the entire sentence through clenched lips. "Patti, we have a change of plans." She planted her purse firmly in the center of her lap. "I'm calling Lizzy in Pittsburgh. You'll go there, have the baby and give it up for adoption. You'll come home, resume your life and it will be like nothing has happened. There are no easy solutions to this problem — but there are solutions."

CHAPTER 15

ALTHOUGH I'D TAKEN THE NIGHT TRAIN to McKeesport with Mom to visit family for as long as I could remember, this time it was Daddy who dropped me off at the train station. As hard as I tried, I couldn't think of a thing to say to him when we were in the car. I think we were both relieved to hear the train whistle. Daddy gave me an awkward pat on the back and mumbled something about remembering to help Lizzy with whatever she needed, and said he'd be in touch. I wanted to hug him hard and tell him not to worry about me, but instead I did what I always did, and patted his back, too.

The train was almost empty so I found a seat next to the window and placed my purse on the seat beside me, hoping I would not have to move it so I wouldn't have to talk to anyone. I must have fallen asleep immediately. I was awakened by the train screeching to a halt to allow a group of coal miners to board; I knew we must be close to McKeesport. The miners all carried identical metal lunch boxes. Except for the occasional grunt or nod, they didn't talk to each other. Some wore overalls. They all wore hard hats, making them look almost like armored warriors. I peered out the window into the darkness. The metallic smell of the dusty train mixed with the beginning streaks of the hazy pumpkin sky, and I thought of Mom and Daddy and Goldie still asleep in their beds at home. I'd never been to Pittsburgh without Mom, and although it was not unfamiliar, this time it was different. I glanced across the aisle at a man, actually a boy who didn't look much older than I. He stared straight ahead, into the back of the neck of the man seated in front of him, and barely moved—not even when the train jerked and creaked to begin again. He looked a little like a statue, and for a moment I wanted to stand up and scream at him that I was pregnant and not married—that I hadn't even gone all the way; that I was barely seventeen, like he was, and I didn't even have a husband. I didn't belong with all these dead eyes and metal lunch boxes.

I unbuttoned my circular Chiquita banana skirt and noticed how one of the bananas seemed to be popping straight out over my stomach where the fabric was pulled. Soft curves had replaced my straight hips. Even my arms and legs looked softer and shapelier. But it was my breasts that fascinated me the most. Sometimes they were sore and bumped into things, like they were in the way. Some days they seemed as though they belonged to someone else. They'd grown so large they spilled out over the new bras Mom had bought me. She warned me to wear the ugly brassieres all the time, never take them off, not even when I slept. She said they would keep me firm, which I guessed would help keep the secret better. It was important to erase all signs of the pregnancy from my body–as though it had never happened. But the truth was that secretly I liked to look at my new breasts when I caught a glimpse of my profile in store windows.

I was traveling to a new place and a new identity. Mom and Lizzy had talked a lot during the last couple of weeks and come up with a plan for me. I was to tell everyone that I had run away and married a soldier who had been sent to Germany. My name was

Patti Steinhoff, Mom's maiden name, and I had come to McKeesport to help Lizzy and attend business school. I liked the idea of having a new self; the old self wasn't working very well.

There was one thing I had to do before leaving home, and I waited until the day before I was to leave to do it. I had to go to the Jewish Social Service Adoption Agency downtown and set up the arrangements for the adoption. Although Mom had done the research and found the agency, she made a surprising decision to let me handle this appointment alone.

I had chosen my clothes carefully, wanting to make sure I made a good impression. I tried to think of it as a job interview as I pulled a pale blue cotton shirtwaist dress from my closet. It buttoned all the way down the front so it hid my thickened waist, if one didn't look from the side. I pulled on a pair of Mom's nylons, checking to make sure the seams were straight, and slipped into a pair of high-heeled pumps. Next I checked my face in the bathroom mirror and noticed it was softer, fuller. I rubbed a little lipstick on my already pink cheeks and took the curlers out of my hair, letting it fall down around my shoulders. I couldn't help but notice that being pregnant made my hair shinier. I dropped the five-dollar bill that Mom had left on the table into my purse and waited on the front porch for the cab to pick me up.

We pulled up in front of an old building in northwest Washington, off of 13th Street, in an area of downtown where I'd never been. The building had a rounded green dome on the rooftop, making it look a little like a castle in a fairy tale. A Jewish star engraved on a brass plaque hung above the door with the words Jewish Social Service Agency written inside of it.

The woman at the desk seemed to be waiting for me. She ushered me into a windowless office where she told me to sit on a folding chair across from a messy desk piled with manila folders. She told me that a caseworker would be in shortly. It was the first time I'd heard the term "caseworker." I kind of liked the idea of having my own person assigned to me.

A short, platinum-haired woman with brilliant red finger-nails and a husky voice that sounded almost like a man's walked in and closed the door. She motioned for me to stay seated. When she smiled, she reminded me of the school nurse when I pretend-ed to have monthly cramps, but was really trying to get out of class—like she knew something I didn't, but was going to be nice anyway.

"Hello, Patti. My name is Madeleine Greenberg and I'll be working with you during your confinement. Your mother has kindly filled me in on many of the, umm, details, of your situation and I'm sure we can be friends."

She had a tiny diamond ring on her pinkie finger and when she saw me notice it she sat up a little straighter. It was then, I made the decision to dislike her. She extended her hand, and for a minute I was reminded of a parrot. Her red fingers looked like claws.

"Nice to meet you," I said, standing up to shake her hand. It was suddenly enormously important that I impress her.

"Are you sure this is what you want to do?" she said, listen-ing too hard—like she didn't already know the answer. "Your baby will be given to a wonderful family."

I wondered why everybody always referred to these people as a "wonderful family." I didn't understand how anyone knew they were wonderful, since nobody even knew them yet.

"You know you're doing a very unselfish thing by allowing your child to grow up in a home where he will be loved and taken care of by people who desperately want a child. Your baby will be given opportunities that you can never provide. We take great care in matching our babies up with families who share similar back-grounds."

I was struck by the word "our." My baby isn't "ours," I thought. It's mine. It was the first time I had felt anything even bordering on ownership of my child, and I physically pulled away from her. It dawned on me that this woman was going to take my baby away.

She went on to explain that confidentiality would be completely honored, and that once I signed the papers, I would never, ever be able to see my baby again; nor would the adoptive parents ever know my identity. She'd already said this more than once; why did she have to repeat it? Where do they hide these papers, I thought, and who guarded them? I tried to concentrate on Madeleine Greenberg's words, but instead, I thought how she would look holding a baby. Her long fingernails would probably scratch it. I wondered what the baby's adoptive mother would look like, if she'd have red hair like me.

Madeleine droned on, asking me questions about my interests and hobbies. She wanted to know about Daddy and his violin playing. She even said she'd try and match the baby up with a family who liked music. Who doesn't like music? But then she asked if it were at all possible to speak to the birth father to get a family history from him. I remembered Robert's offer to "do anything" and I felt something inside of me wake up. I knew he hadn't yet left for Texas, and somehow, it felt good to know he'd have to come here, too — like he really was a part of this.

"Oh, yes," I said. "He'll do anything I ask him to. We'd be married right now, if things had just been a little different. He's very much in love with me; it just didn't work out."

"I'm sure he cared about you," Madeleine said, but it was obvious she didn't believe it at all. She reached over to pat my hand, and I pulled it back. She handed me a card with her name printed in gold.

"Give him my number and we'll set up a meeting after you've left for Pittsburgh. We'll keep in touch with your mom during your absence and set everything else up for the last month before the birth."

I was in such a hurry to get out of her office that I stumbled on my high heels.

I told no one about the phone call to Robert, but it's the last thing I did before I left. I called his parents' home where he answered. The call was terse. He listened long enough for me to read Madeleine Greenberg's name to him. When he answered that yes, he'd go, I felt relieved. After I hung up, there was one more thing to do: I hid his senior class picture inside my wallet behind my identification card.

By the time the train pulled into McKeesport, my headache was better and I'd almost forgotten the coal miners.

Lizzy and Morrie had been a part of my life forever. Like Ninny and Uncle Charlie and Ruth, they had always been there. The difference was that they stayed in Pittsburgh and didn't migrate to Maryland like the rest of the family. Everyone had always tried to get them to move, but I guessed they had their reasons, because they stayed. For a time it seemed like they had made the best decision, because Morrie had apparently gotten a traveling salesman job selling aluminum siding to people who lived out in the country. Uncle Lenny, one of Mom's favorite cousins, hired him for a while. Mom was convinced they had all become gangsters when they all bought big black Cadillacs. She said she couldn't recognize any of them any more. I remembered how she'd spent lots of time on the phone with Lizzy giving advice. I guessed it didn't last too long, because pretty soon there was a big scandal, and Uncle Lenny had to go to jail for a while. Mom said it wasn't really jail, more a country club, and besides, Uncle Lenny got to lose weight. For a while everyone thought that Morrie might have to go to jail too, but he proclaimed loudly to anyone who would listen that he was not a "closer," which apparently meant he did nothing wrong. I guessed just the closers got in trouble. All I knew was Uncle Lenny was about as much of a gangster as Jackie Gleason. He one of the sweetest, gentlest people I'd ever known. So, by the time I went to live with them, they weren't rich any more.

The conductor put my suitcase on the platform and helped me down the train steps. I felt the strongest urge to get back on the train and just keep going. I'd never really spent any time alone with Morrie and Lizzy, and here I was moving into their house. I had no idea what I would say when I saw them.

Lizzy's carrot-red hair stood out against the gray morning. She was waving at me so hard that she lost her grip on Donnie, her seven-year-old, who was wandering too close to the moving train. I waved back, feeling stupid because it already felt like we were all trying too hard. I was glad when she stopped to grab Donnie by his collar to pull him back to safety. Little Lainey, who I thought was about nine, was hanging back, eyeing me like she was wondering why I was there. She had tight little black curls that sprung out from her small head like macaroni and enormous black eyes that made no attempt to mask her curiosity. She was, for some unknown reason, always known as Little Lainey. The first thing I noticed as I walked toward them was Lizzy's belly. She was skinny as a stick except for her protruding tummy, which was already the size of a small watermelon. I struggled to keep my eyes on her face and not stare. Both of our babies were due in October, but I figured she was bigger because it was her third kid, and she'd already got a head start on stretching. Lizzy was more like Mom's age, and quick to tell everyone in the family that her pregnancy was definitely not planned. She gave me a quick hug and told me Morrie was in the car waiting and we were all going to Solly's deli for breakfast. I had no idea who Solly was, but I figured I should know him, so I acted like I did. Turned out he was Morrie's brother. Apparently Morrie had lots of brothers and sisters, and they all lived within a couple of miles of each other.

Morrie motioned for us to get in—actually got out of the car and opened the back door for me. He helped me into the back seat, where I wedged myself in between the kids.

Little Lainey, who had hardly taken her eyes off of me for a second, finally blurted out, "You don't look fat like Mommy. Where's your baby? I can't even see it inside your tummy. Can I feel?"

Lizzy gently grabbed her little girl by the arm and told her to stop bothering me, but Little Lainey continued to stare at me, like I was a tourist attraction. I didn't know why I did it, but I took her hand and laid it on my stomach. I couldn't really think of anything to say, but this seemed to calm her, and me too. I liked the feel of her chubby little hand as she moved closer to me, even snuggled her head on my shoulder.

Nobody ever asked me about Robert or even mentioned that I was having his baby. They sure made a big deal out of Lizzy's baby, though. Morrie came in every night and put his ear to her tummy like he was talking on a telephone. He said stuff like "hello in there, this is your father"…and then pretended the baby answered. Maybe they were all afraid they'd hurt my feelings if they said anything funny to me, since she got to keep her baby and I didn't.

Little Lainey was the only one too young to be polite. After we were in bed at night she snuggled up beside me in the twin beds we'd pushed together. Lizzy made sure I got the spot by the window, and told the kids I needed more room. Little Lainey slept in the middle, next to me, and Donnie was on the end, but mostly on the floor. Little Lainey liked to touch my belly before she went to sleep. She'd always pat it with a gentle force, as if it were the shell of a soft-boiled egg. She always asked what the baby's name was. I

Good Girls Don't

made up crazy names like Bartholomew or Garbanzo Bean or Olaf, and I'd fall asleep giggling. These were the best times of my day.

Little Lainey and I were lying in bed together when I felt the baby move for the first time. It was just a twitch, and at first I thought it was gas, but after the third time, I knew it was him. Somehow I knew it was not a her, though I don't know how. He felt like a tiny sparrow fluttering his wings in a place so deep inside of me that I had never even known it existed. For a moment everything vanished except that spot, and I forgot to breathe for a long time. I almost woke Little Lainey so she could feel it too, but changed my mind, and lay there waiting for another twitch, until the sun came up.

After that I began to fall into the routine of the household, actually relaxed a little. I stopped thinking there was something I should be doing. Lizzy played mahjong every Wednesday night with her girlfriends while Morrie went to the American Legion Hall with his brothers. Lizzy and her friends sat around a card table in the living room and mostly gossiped and ate bologna sandwiches, and talked about their husbands. I pretended to hang around for the food, but the truth was, I liked to listen to their stories. They were all much older than me; two of them were pregnant, and they all had kids. It was the first time I'd been included in a group of grown-up women who talked about everything to each other. I liked being treated like one of them, even though they didn't talk much to me.

I was especially lonely on mahjong nights. The women made me wish I had a husband, too. Mostly I was aware of the beginnings of a conflicted wish that I could keep my baby. I wasn't exactly sure when he stopped being a grapefruit, and became my baby, but he did. Maybe it was after I felt his little elbow actually lift my tummy a little. I wasn't sure if it was his elbow or his knee, but for a minute it felt a little like he was in my arms.

The tiny house trapped the heat inside like a furnace. The only relief was a small electric fan that everyone in the house fought over, but that usually stayed in Lizzy and Morrie's bedroom. I didn't mind because it drowned out the sounds. The walls were so thin that I could practically hear them breathe. It wasn't like I heard sex noises, just whispers. When Morrie came home late one night from the American Legion, I actually heard him pull down the covers and ask Lizzy if he could just "touch her there for a minute." I heard the swish of her nightgown as I imagined him lifting it over her head. I thought I heard her giggle. I didn't know if I actually heard the nightgown, but it sounded like it to me. It made me wish it were Robert's hand on my belly, not Little Lainey's.

Mom arranged for me to attend business school during my exile. We both agreed it would give me something else to think about and help pass the time. Douglas Business School was above Langley Cafeteria on Main Street in downtown McKeesport. Next door to it was a furniture store with couches in the window, all covered in plastic, like the one in Lizzy's living room, and on the other side was one of a dozen bars sprinkled throughout the town. The American Legion Hall was on Hadley Street, right across from the bus stop, and the movie theater was at the end of the block. It was a great theater, left over from vaudeville, with an upstairs balcony almost bigger than the Capitol Theater in Washington. I guessed McKeesport had a lot of Catholics because St. Michael's Church was the biggest building in town. Busy, too. I always saw people going in and out. I guessed that Catholics had to pray a lot. Mom said that Jews could go into their closets and God would hear them, but Catholics always had to make a big deal out of everything.

Years of coal dust had settled into every crease and corner of life in this town, leaving everything a dull gray. I straightened my

Good Girls Don't

new white top, which the dust had already begun to dim, and climbed the two flights of stairs to the school. I practiced saying my new name, Mrs. Max Steinhoff. That was Mom's father's name. I made a bold decision before I reached the top of the stairs.

"Hi" I said much too brightly to a woman seated behind a desk. "I'm Mrs. Robert Steinhoff." The name even shocked me. But, there it was, Robert Steinhoff. I had to chuckle to myself at the combination of Mom's maiden name, mixed with Robert. Now that's a strange couple. I was so excited by the new name, I followed it up with far more information than the lady asked for.

"I'm here staying with family while my husband is stationed in Germany. He's in the army, you know. He wanted me to go with him in the worst way, but we thought, under the circumstances," I paused, looking innocently at my tummy, slightly touching it, "we thought this was better for everyone. I needed something to do to keep me entertained while he's gone. I can't imagine that I'll ever have to use it, but shorthand sounds kinda interesting."

The lady at the desk never looked up, just hunted in a small index box and pulled out a card that said Patti Steinhoff, and told me to take a seat in the first classroom on the left.

For months all I'd thought about was the pregnancy. Mom, of course, lived it morning noon and night, and if there was any time left over, it was more than filled by Daddy's silence. Just avoiding my friends took up the rest. So, when I entered a place where nobody really cared all that much about me, I was frankly a little shocked. People either believed me, or they didn't, but for sure nobody really cared very much. It was the first time I was left to carve out my own days. Free to have thoughts, create fantasies, or, as it turned out, to tell elaborate lies.

The class was filled with young girls, most of whom were there either because they had flunked something in school, or because their parents wanted them doing something more productive than hanging out at the swimming pool to meet boys. The girls taking shorthand that summer were clearly not there because they wanted to be. Taking summer school business classes was nothing that anyone in their right mind would choose to do if they had a choice. So, when I walked into the class, my belly gave me immediate status. I didn't have to do anything to be unique. I took a seat toward the back and pretended to study the shorthand book as though I was reading a novel. A few of the girls actually turned around and openly stared at me. For the first time I felt a strange comfort in being pregnant. I didn't have to be pretty, or even interested in boys. I couldn't compete with them, so I didn't have to be anything—except pregnant.

I'd replaced everything that used to be me with a lie. When the teacher called my name, Patti Steinhoff, for roll call, I answered in a voice so strong and clear I barely recognized it. The morning passed quickly. The little squiggly shorthand lines began to have meaning, and for a while I was engrossed. When lunch was called I grabbed my paper bag with a salami sandwich and a fresh peach that I'd packed earlier that morning, and began to head down the hall to the lunchroom. I took a seat by the window, fully prepared to continue studying while I ate. But I was soon interrupted by two girls, who had taken the seats on the long bench beside me.

"Hi," said the one with the large face and firm features. She snapped her butter-blonde ponytail with a practiced flick of her head and announced her name, as though it were a title. "I'm Victoria. You're not from around here, are you?"

"No, " I shrugged. "I'm from Washington, D.C. I'm staying with family for the summer." It was easier to say D.C. I heard the girl on the other side of me tear open a bag of potato chips, and turned just in time to see her small perfect teeth rip the package open. Her eyes never left me while she devoured the chips in two handfuls.

"My name is Patti," I said, choosing to leave out Steinhoff.

Apparently we weren't using last names, and the new one was still a bit hard to get out. It had only been hours before that I'd given myself Robert's name. It was one thing to pronounce it to a faceless clerk, but I wasn't yet ready to say it to these two.

The potato chip girl stared without blinking. "Joanne," she said, her small brown eyes focused in on me like a ferret. "I'm Joanne." She glanced down at the near-empty bag and thrust it in front of me. "Here," she said, "have one."

I reached in and took out the last of a few crumbly potato chips and thanked her.

"So why in the world would anyone come to McKeesport if they didn't have to," Jessica said. "Jeez, all we wanna do is get outta here."

"Well, my hubby got sent off to Munich, Germany. He's in the Air Force, so we decided it would be better for me to wait out the baby here. I'm staying with my Mom's cousin. She's pregnant too, so we thought it'd be kinda fun to be together. Being we're both going to have babies at the same time and everything." Once I started I couldn't stop. It was like stuff had been stored up forever, just waiting to pour out. I couldn't have found two better listeners than Victoria and Joanne. The harder they listened, the more I talked.

"Rob, that's what I call him. His name is really Robert, but my special name for him is Rob. He's a pilot—" and then I added, "and an officer. We're going to move to Texas as soon as he comes home. But, for sure, he'll be home in time for the baby in October. They're giving him special leave."

For just a second, I thought of Robert already in Texas with his new pregnant wife, Mitzi. I wondered if she was bigger than I was and if her baby was moving around inside of her, like mine. For a second I allowed myself to wonder if he even thought of me at all. If sometimes he looked at her and wished it were me—

maybe one day he'd wonder why his baby didn't look like me.

I quickly got rid of the thought and paused for a minute, to look kindly at my audience, like someone imparting precious information.

"Wow," Joanne uttered, chomping on a tuna fish sandwich with the same amount of force as she had applied to the chips. "You look so young to have to go through all this alone. I could never do that," she added wistfully.

"Me neither, said Victoria, who, by now looked less regal. "You're really brave to come here. It must be really hard."

"Oh, it's not that hard. I just try and think about Rob. Poor baby, he's the one who has it tough. I mean Munich, Germany is pretty dangerous. We don't like to think of what could happen over there."

I realized I might have gone a little too far with that last remark. After all, we were not at war with anyone, and I couldn't think of anything very dangerous going on in Germany.

But apparently, Victoria and Joanne were far more interested in romance than politics, because it went right over them.

"We were in school together. Rob was three years older, really popular, and we just couldn't stay away from one another. We just had to be together. We ran off to Baltimore while he was in college and eloped."

By this time both girls were glued to me, their eyes soft and dreamy, as though I were reading from a romance novel. I was actually sorry when the bell rang for us to return to the classroom

After that, there were days when I almost believed I was Mrs. Robert Steinhoff. I wrote the name all over my shorthand book, signed all my papers in oversized handwriting that didn't even resemble my usual tight, cramped signature, and always referred to my husband as Rob. My stories were peppered with "poor baby" or "sweet hubby." I had no idea where these stupid names came from. For sure, I never heard them in my home. It was kind of like being taken over by someone else's fantasies—someone I didn't even like very much. By the time I realized that I could barely find myself inside all the lies, I'd already become the class celebrity.

One afternoon, late in July, I returned home from school to find Little Lainey waiting on the front stoop, her eyes sparkling so brightly they were about to leap out of her head.

"You got an important letter," she crowed with joy. "Mommy won't tell me who it's from, but I bet I know. It's Garbanzo Bean's Daddy, I just know it."

Little Lainey led me up to the bedroom where the letter was propped up against my pillow, and when I saw my name sprawled in black ink across the envelope, the possibility that it was from Robert made me dizzy.

"Is it from him? Is it the baby's Daddy? What did he say? C'mon, read it to me," said Lainey, her eyes pleading.

"No," I answered, "it's not from him. I won't be hearing from him."

"You don't know that," she said, and headed downstairs.

I lay on the bed and watched the afternoon sun filter through the Venetian blinds lighting up the letter with golden stripes. When I finally opened it and saw that it was from Ralph, there was a sense of relief.

Dear Patti,

I had to really work your Mom to get your address. I don't know what all the secrecy is about but you sure left town in a cloud of dust. I tried to see you lots of times after you left the hospital but your Mom was guarding you like a Brinks truck. No offense to your Mom, I'm sure she had her reasons. I don't want you to think I'm prying, but I want you to know I'm here for you if you just want to talk about anything -- anything!!!! There's nothing you can't tell me that I won't understand. If you're in any kind of trouble or if you just want to talk, I'm here.

I wanted you to know I'm off to NYU next year, but I couldn't leave Maryland without letting you know. I think you're a great girl with a wonderful mind and you're cute as a button. I could never get the nerve up to tell you this, but you were the best part of Maryland University for me. I'm not sure what's going on, and it's definitely not my business, but I want you to know you have a friend who thinks you're great, no matter what.

Love,
Ralph

I put the letter down and for a minute listened to the sounds of the kids playing tag outside the open window. Little Lainey was "it" and their giggles floated up into the bedroom sounding like a litter of puppies. I took in Ralph's words and let them remind me of the sweet evenings we had spent together, when we told each other everything. I was struck by how far I'd come in my impersonation of myself. I imagined Ralph's practical voice telling me to shape up and stop being such a goofball. Just then the baby kicked a nudge, like he was reminding me that he, too, agreed with Ralph.

That night, in bed, I lay very still on my back, my hands over the top of my belly, waiting for a sign that my baby was awake. He usually let me know with a long, sleepy stretch-like he was turning over. I could almost hear him yawn. I loved these gentle turns the best. These were the ones that filled me up like I'd just eaten Thanksgiving dinner and wanted to lie on the couch and stare at nothing. Some nights he swam and played—let me know he was quite happy to be in my tummy. Other nights he jabbed and punched to let me know he wanted to talk. I tried to imagine what he would look like at three, or when he began school. I wondered if he would ever think of me, or wonder what I looked like—and if he'd hate asparagus like I did. I wondered if he'd be good at math, or be skinny, or big like Robert.

"I hope Mitzi is big and fat and ugly by now," I said, patting him. "You know, if your Daddy hadn't done it with her we'd be married now and I'd be living in Texas with him. But I don't want you to worry," I added quickly, "because Madeleine Greenberg is looking for the best home in the whole world for you. Just because she has that funny voice and I didn't like her much, doesn't mean she doesn't know her job. Besides, you don't have to be with her for long, just enough time to get you to the right Mommy and Daddy who can give you stuff. By the time you remember any-thing you'll wake up in a perfect baby room with a beautiful Mommy who will rock you in an old rocking chair that has prob-ably been in her family for years. She'll probably look like Maureen O'Hara, with long red hair. It'll be a wonderful family."

The next day after school I didn't go right home, but decided to take a walk through town by myself. I crossed Hadley Street and went down Baker and passed a group of boys hanging on the cor-ner, who looked up at me as I passed, but quickly looked away when they saw my belly. They went back to their girl-watching, and I continued down Baker. It felt good to walk, to do whatever I wanted for a change. I didn't know what I'd do, but I was excited to be alone, moving down a new street, looking at something dif-ferent. I climbed a steep unfamiliar hill lined with storefronts already preparing for closing. I passed a man and woman holding hands, walking together at a leisurely pace, leaning in toward each other, backlit by the soft creamy glow of the afternoon sun. He said something to her and she laughed.

I was alone, I thought, as the couple disappeared around the corner. The world suddenly seemed distant, and I felt larger, clumsier actually, than everything around me. The excitement of the adventure I had felt just seconds ago moved on. It didn't vanish, just simply moved through me, and floated out of sight. Maybe if I walked faster I would find the good feeling again. Right now I couldn't look back, but must continue walking. The bells from the Catholic Church rang out loudly as I walked to their rhythm, like a metronome. I passed a bus stop and remembered I'd missed my bus, but recklessly continued on, choosing not to call Lizzy. I knew I'd have to wait another hour for the next bus, but I didn't mind. It felt right to be a little lost today.

"We have a whole hour to do whatever we want," I said silently to the baby. "Let's pretend we're in London, England, and we're going to meet your Daddy. He's the son of a Count but he's so in love with me, and thinks I'm so beautiful, that he's going to give up his royal future to run away with me. His family doesn't approve of us, but we don't care. I'll bet he has a big bunch of roses for us when we see him. He always likes to bring us flowers. Would you like to have an English Daddy who talks like he's in the movies? Or maybe we could be in Paris, France, and spend the afternoon having a picnic by the Seine, while we wait for your Daddy to join us. He's handsome and sings French songs. Even knows French lullabies that he's going to teach us."

I was so lost in my daydreams I didn't notice the massive granite building that seemed to have sprung up right in front of me. The chime, now distant, rang as I stopped in front of the wide curved steps directly in front of the etched letters over the door that spelled out *McKeesport Public Library*. There was no hesitation

Good Girls Don't

as I entered, as though it'd been my destination since the beginning. The musty comfort was immediate. I even liked the crisp sound my sandals made on the marble floor, announcing my arrival to a white-haired lady dressed in black, behind the dark wood counter. Her smile welcomed me as though she'd been waiting for me all day. I dragged my hand along the polished mahogany table that stood by the entrance, and let my gaze wander across the stacks of books piled neatly in its center. I reached for one of the books that had fallen on its side, apart from the others, and read the title: *The Brothers Karamazov*, by Dostoevsky.

I opened the book to somewhere near the middle and began to read. Although the language was strange, the words pulled me into a world so compelling that once I'd begun, I felt duty bound to continue. I couldn't understand these characters or even pronounce their strange-sounding names, but it didn't matter, because the music of the language of this village in Russia soothed me in a way that nothing else ever had. A place opened up inside me that up until now had remained closed. I had to read a page over several times to fully understand it, but in the quiet, I forgot the boys on the corner who looked away when I passed, and the couple who made me feel lonely.

When finally I looked up from the book, I noticed a young mother sitting at a table across the room with a child about five or six. She was pointing at a book and whispering something to him that I couldn't hear. Even the little boy seemed aware of the agreement to be still. It was as though everyone in the room had entered into a state of reverence, even awe. I liked how the thick book felt in my hands, and tucked it under my arm with a rare assurance. I promised myself I would read this, finish it, no matter how long it took, or how hard I would have to struggle to understand it. I knew somehow that by doing this I'd become connected to a deeper part of myself. It was in the quiet of the library that the cacophony of voices (Mom, Daddy, even Robert) that usually crowded my head gradually faded, and I felt myself bonding with myself and, because he was there, with my baby.

CHAPTER 16

The first pain was swift and sharp. It was familiar, like the stab from an arrow flung across time and buried deep inside the souls of all women.

THE OCTOBER NIGHT WAS BLACK; the sky was empty, starless. I looked for the moon but all I saw was a sliver of orange. Ninny knew right away that it was time. She took the dishtowel from my hand and ordered me to go into her bedroom and lie down on the bed. I lay on the soft double bed that smelled of sweet tobacco and lavender soap, the one Ninny shared with Uncle Charlie. I pulled the pink afghan up around my chin. I stared at the ceiling, and wished it were over. Streaks of light from the lamp made shadows on the ceiling that squirmed over my head, like wingless angels.

My belly was still. It no longer rolled and kicked from side to side. It felt heavy, like a stone held inside of a peach. The pain jabbed, slammed into my back. I yelled, even though I didn't want to. Soon Mom was lying beside me. She laid me on my side and held my hard belly with her small, warm hands.

"Soon, Patti, soon," she crooned over and over.

Soon I'd be able to sleep in my own bed, and see Patsy, and wear normal clothes. I'd never have to see Madeleine Greenberg again, or listen to her tell me about my baby's wonderful new family. I was sick of her weekly visits, telling me how unselfish I was, and how I was making another family so happy. I didn't care a bit about that other family.

I heard Ninny tell Uncle Charlie in the other room, "Forget your Masonic meeting tonight. You have to drive her. Laura says they'll take a cab but I don't think so. And leave your pipe here, the smell makes her sick."

Mom sure got there fast. I was sure she didn't tell the Yellow Cab Company why she needed one right away, she was so careful about making sure nobody suspected anything. Ninny always said Mom should have been a lawyer, but I thought she should have been a CIA agent.

It had been decided that I would return back to Maryland and go into hiding at Ninny and Uncle Charlie's apartment during the last month of my pregnancy. Since I'd returned from Pittsburgh Mom had been different. She came over to Ninny's almost every night to see me. We walked around the apartment complex, talked about all kinds of stuff—Goldie's dance recital and Patsy's new boyfriend—not just about me being pregnant. Lately she'd even brought me Hershey bars—broke off a piece or two and handed it to me, while we walked. I guessed she understood how living here had been like prison. I was so fat that Dr. Cohen had made me eat salt-free bread because salt made me retain water. Mom made Ninny watch everything I ate, and I was always hungry. Some days I felt like one of the girls I'd seen in old movies about the war who would do almost anything for a piece of chocolate or nylons. Lately I'd been dreaming about wearing stockings, and high heels, and dressy dresses like I used to wear at dances, instead of the big over-sized coat of Ninny's that I could barely button. I could never go out without her dark green, flowered old lady's babushka. Mom insisted I put on this disguise in case someone recognized me. I had

Good Girls Don't

to wear the same stupid outfit every time Uncle Charlie drove me to the doctor. Once I actually did see Nancy Atkins crossing Georgia Avenue with some boy and had to duck down in the car, even with the disguise. I told Mom I probably called more attention to myself in this get-up than walking down Georgia Avenue naked.

The pains were coming faster now. Mom's hand on my belly felt cool. She was rubbing it at the same time she was holding her wristwatch underneath the lamp by the bed.

"It's time to call Sidney."

Mom had switched from the soft croon to her take-over voice. I liked her hand on my belly. I didn't want her to leave to go to the phone.

"They're about fifteen minutes apart. I'm sure he'll want us to leave now."

Mom dialed the number that she'd obviously memorized.

"Please have the Doctor call me immediately," she ordered. She called out Ninny's phone number slowly, drawing out her words. "Patti is in labor. It's time."

I noticed as we got into Uncle Charlie's car that the tiny crescent of orange moon had slipped completely out of sight. Ninny's gray woolen coat lay open across my belly. Once again I sat in the back seat of his car, my head beginning to ache from Mom's Fabergé perfume. This time we were not on our way to Baltimore to get rid of the baby; we were going to the hospital to have the baby. But we were still going to get rid of it. I didn't want to think about that. I wondered if they would put me to sleep, and when I awoke the baby would simply disappear and I'd be back home like none of this had ever happened. My head was throbbing from the perfume but I didn't care. Mom's hand felt firm on my belly. She cradled it like she had the power to keep the baby safely inside of me, a while longer.

Another jab. This time it lingered, like a flame bursting down my back, lapping at the sides of my torso. A moan escaped with my breath and Mom immediately groaned with me— soft and low like a hurt kitten. Her sound soothed me, as though we shared the labor. She looked at me closely, examined my face as if she'd never seen it before. She twined her fingers into mine like we used to when I was little and had played the game of *Here's the church and here's the steeple.*

"You'll get over this, Patti," she said. "We'll both get over this. I promise you it will be like it never happened. You're smart and after this you'll be even smarter. You'll go on to have other children, and a husband who respects you, and this will become a distant memory."

She pressed my palm down and stroked my fingers. "We're doing the right thing. I'm sure of it," she repeated. "You may be giving up a child, but I'm giving up my grandchild. Don't forget that."

I felt a jolt of anger when she said this, but nodded. My face felt hot and flushed. I didn't want her to talk any more, only to hold me, so I wouldn't hurt. But her dark gaze wouldn't leave my eyes, even when I looked away.

"Yes," I said, in deference to her gaze. "It's the right thing."

I barely got out the words when the next stab of pain came, and Mom tightened her arm around my shoulder until it went away.

Uncle Charlie let us off at the emergency room entrance. A slender young man in a white lab coat was waiting for us with a wheelchair. There was no time for good-byes because I was quickly wheeled down a long corridor. I turned around to find Mom, but we were moving so fast she had already disappeared behind a tall column. Her perfume was quickly replaced by the bitter scents of Clorox and iodine.

I lay on a hard cot inside a stark cubicle, enclosed by a white muslin screen attached to steel rollers. My eyes rested on the screen as I sank into a pain-free moment. I imagined that this was over, and that it was next year, and the year after. I thought of my baby — saw him wearing a birthday hat surrounded by his beautiful redheaded Mommy and strong, loving Daddy. Everyone was looking at the baby, who was smiling and putting his stubby baby fists into a huge chocolate birthday cake. There were presents, lots of them, but I couldn't put a face on the baby. All of a sudden nothing was more important to me than seeing his face — my baby's face. I wanted this more than anything I'd ever wanted, but all I saw was an empty space where his face should be. The pains were coming again, but this time, they didn't hurt as much, because I was searching my mind so hard for a glimpse of my baby's face. A nurse came in and rubbed my forehead; she must have heard me crying.

"You've got a while to go, honey. Your doctor isn't here yet, but someone will be in shortly to examine you," she said, as she wrapped my fingers around the sides of the bars that she was pulling up, like a baby crib.

"Where's my Mom?" I cried. "Tell her to please come in."

"Someone will be along shortly," she repeated.

I didn't believe her. I lay like this for a long time, waiting for Dr. Cohen to come and take the baby. A woman was wheeled past my cubicle. I heard someone scream on the other side of the muslin curtain. No, no, I will not do that, I thought. Then another pain — and another — and another. Soon there was nothing but pain.

"Mom," I cried. "Mom!"

I didn't care who heard me. A different nurse came in. She was fat and had little pig eyes. I hated her. She said it wouldn't be long. I didn't believe her. I was so tired. Why did they lie to me about everything? I pleaded with them to let Mom in. She'd know what to do. I wanted to see my baby's face. I wanted my mother.

Then the doctor was there; someone gave me a shot, and every-thing went black.

When I awoke I was tucked into a hospital bed with the sheets tightly pulled up around me; I could barely move my arms. All I saw was my reflection in Dr. Cohen's horn-rimmed glasses. He was patting me on the head.

"It's all over now and you're as good as new."

I wanted to pull away from him but had nowhere to move. I looked around me, but it was as though I was seeing everything through thick dust. If I didn't answer him maybe I could disappear into the soft pillow. I closed my eyes but couldn't rest.

Who am I? I was so tired of pretending not to love Robert. I wanted to marry him, to know that everything was fine. I wanted to see my baby. I'd thought for so long that after the baby was born everything would go back to the way it used to be. To a time when I knew Robert loved me, when…

"Is he a boy?" I asked, my eyes squeezed tight.

Dr. Cohen kept stroking my head and repeating, "it's all over now."

"Is he a boy?" I repeated, looking right through my reflec-tion into his face. There was something stronger in my voice that made him turn away.

"Yes, it's a boy and he's healthy, 7 pounds 6 ounces," he said. "But, Patti, " he continued, "I don't think it's wise to give you too many details. Remember, we discussed this. Your mother and the social worker, we all feel it will be better if you don't see the baby." My throat tightened.

"Ultimately, it's your decision, of course, but your Mom felt, and we all agreed: you have a long life ahead of you. This will all be a distant memory. I know this isn't easy, dear."

I just stared up into the ceiling, away from his face.

"Maybe next time," he continued, "you'll think a little longer

Good Girls Don't

before you let some boy get all worked up in the back seat of a car. But you're a good girl; I know you'll put this behind you. Forget it. I mean, of course, you won't actually forget it, but it'll just be easier this way."

Finally, he was finished and then he was gone. I lay back on the bed and put my hands on the place where my baby had been only yesterday. Now it felt hollow, empty. Where were the tiny knees and elbows that had become part of me? The skin that stretched over my stomach was no longer taut; instead it was soft and wrinkled like something old. I kept pressing my belly, even though I knew he was no longer there. I couldn't stop searching for him.

A hospital volunteer, barely older than me, wearing a candy-striped red and white uniform, heard my cries, and peeked into the room. Seeing her, I stopped my tears, hardened my voice.

"Take me to the nursery," I pleaded.

She said nothing, but nodded and grabbed a wheelchair from the hallway and helped me into it. She pushed me into the elevator, and for the first time I realized I wasn't on the maternity ward.

"Where am I?"

"You're on the cardiac floor, " she answered. "We shouldn't be doing this. I could get into a lot of trouble. But, I know how you feel. I sure wanted to see my Ellie right away after she was born. Promise not to tell."

I nodded in agreement.

As soon as we got off the elevator I felt my stomach knot. Two black nurses, giggling like schoolgirls approached us. Their laughter exploded as they got closer. A young man holding a bouquet of pink carnations hurried past us, and ducked into a room at the end of the hall. I felt as though we'd walked into a party instead of a hospital ward. The two nurses abruptly stopped laughing when the young candy striper stopped them and whispered something in their ears. I heard only muted sounds that suggested uncertainty. They looked at me, but only for a second, before averting their eyes. The older of the two, a large square-jawed woman, her slick, ebony hair pushed carelessly into a net, finally spoke to me.

"Are you sure you want to do this, young lady?" she asked, not unkindly. "We were told you didn't want to see him, so we've been givin' him extra attention all day. But it's your decision. Nobody can stop you from seein' your own child. I mean, you're the one that's been laying up there for fourteen hours havin' him. The Lord didn't mean for nobody else to see him first, if you don't want them to. Hmmmph! It sure ain't no picnic havin' babies, and if you want to hold that little gift from God nobody should stop it. That's how I see it, anyway. And I'm the one in charge here today, so I'm makin' the decisions. You got that, Daisy?"

She looked hard at the younger girl standing quietly beside her. Daisy's purple earbobs danced around her face as she nodded in agreement.

"You just sit tight there, little lady, and I'll go fetch him for you."

She spun around and marched down the hall to the nurses' station, slipping out of sight, and reappearing almost immediately holding a baby in a blue fuzzy blanket resting inside of arms that looked as though they were constructed specifically for the purpose of baby holding. She placed my child into the crook of my arms.

I pulled back the corner of the blanket, rested his head inside the palm of my hand and stared into the face of my son. He was wrinkled and pink. His eyes fluttered and opened, and then he squeezed them shut again. It was almost as though he was not quite ready to face this world. I wanted to tell him I felt that way, too. I traced his perfectly shaped ears with my finger.

Good Girls Don't

"I'll never, ever forget you, my sweet baby boy," I whispered. "Even when I'm really old—and you're old. I promise every October to remember."

When I leaned down to kiss his heart-shaped lips, I nuzzled my face into his neck and drew in his sweet baby scent. Then I laid him on my lap and lifted the thin cotton blanket away from his body, and examined his fingers and toes. I became lost in the perfection of his miniature nail beds, so smooth and complete. I clutched his warm little body against mine, and rubbed my hands over his back, over his brand new skin, until finally, I handed him back to the nurse. I watched as she scurried down the long hospital corridor with my baby hidden inside her arms. When she turned the corner, a wisp of blue blanket fluttered like the wings of a bird.

I shivered uncontrollably, and then something cracked deep inside my chest where he had just been. My sobs startled me; they were noisy and violent, and seemed to come directly from the void in my belly.

CHAPTER 17

JUST BEFORE THANKSGIVING, WITH ONE DECADE preparing to slip into another, I was fiercely attempting to pretend that the previous year had never happened. Although the starched and crinolined prom dresses still hung in my closet and Eisenhower was still President, I knew that life for me was forever changed. The night that Mom had pronounced me ready to re-enter the world and return home, I was so happy to resume my old life that for a day or two I almost forgot the previous nine months.

I pulled Mom's baggy sweater over my full breasts and made sure it fell low enough to hide the gaping zipper of my skirt. Ninny stood at the doorway to her apartment and waved at me as I silently followed Daddy out to the car. We avoided talking much during the short ride home from Ninny's apartment, but I was so grateful to shed Ninny's flowered scarf and oversized coat I hardly noticed. I opened the car window and stuck my head out into the cool autumn morning. My hair blew straight back, making me feel clean and new again. I was reminded of one of Mom's family stories about my great-grandmother. This must be the way she felt when she arrived in this country, with her hair defiantly bobbed. Apparently she had thrown her obligatory wig, worn by old-world Jewish wives in those days, overboard, during her trip from Hungary to America. I, too, was tossing away a defunct identity. By the time we turned onto Cleveland Avenue and I caught sight of the big oak tree that stood in the front yard exactly where it had always been, all the months of fear and anguish turned into relief. The reassuring oak leaves whirling in small golden piles all over the front yard, just as they did every year, telling me that the ordeal truly was over and I was finally home.

When I caught a glimpse of Goldie, who disappeared behind the white, criss-cross living-room curtains. I jumped out of the car, taking the three steps up our front porch in one leap, and pushed open the door into a world where every formerly familiar thing that was always ordinary became blindingly extraordinary. My little sister, who I hadn't seen in months, had been told that I was away at business school in Pittsburgh. We fell into each other's arms as we had never done before. Something in the way she held on to me told me that she knew far more about where I'd been than we were prepared to talk about. I broke away from her but she continued to clutch my waist. "Welcome home, Sissy. I missed you," she said. I rested my head against the top of hers and hugged her back. "Me too," I whispered.

Goldie led me, almost shyly, up the stairs to the closed door of my room. She jumped ahead of me and opened the door with an exaggerated flourish, beckoning me inside. Strips of yellow and green crepe paper had been taped to the ceiling, where they hung in a brilliant fusion of bouncing colored corkscrews that looked like dancing marionettes. The words WELCOME HOME had been printed on a flattened paper bag with every color from the crayon box and Scotch-taped over my bed. Tears stung my face, and when finally they flowed, I thought they would never stop.

The next few days were a jumble of sensations that took me by surprise from moment to moment. Everything was the same and everything was different. The only sign that I had given birth to a child was a thick red scar that traveled from my naval to the top of my pubic bone, where the incision to remove the ovarian cyst had stretched during my pregnancy. But I knew all too well that I was a young woman with a secret, and truthfully, I thought of little else. I wore my secret like a rash; the more I tried to erase the memory, the itchier I got. Mom and I had spent so much time planning the birth, my escape to Pittsburgh, the adoption, that we had not spoken of what was to come after. The only thing for sure was that we would never speak of this episode again.

I was not prepared for the emotional leaps that I was taking from moment to moment. I had been the center of my family's world for almost a year, or at least that's what I believed, and when I found myself spending time alone, no longer counting days or waiting for time to pass, I became oddly lonely. Daddy escaped into Washington society music jobs — the businessman's bounce, as he called it; Mom became the vice president of the Takoma Park Chamber of Commerce; Lizzy gave birth to a beautiful dark-eyed baby girl, a month after I left Pittsburgh; and Patsy was tucked away in the dorm at Maryland University.

As for me, I had no idea what I was supposed to do or, for that matter, be — or even feel. I was envious of anyone who had a place to go. My first day of euphoria quickly changed to boredom and then depression. I knew I didn't want to go back to school -- at least not just yet. I tried to block out the image of that last moment with my baby. It was over and I needed to forget. Mom had certainly made that clear to me. But the images of him were always lingering somewhere close, surfacing when I least expect- ed it. Who was holding him? Did his eyes stay blue? What did his new mother look like? Did he have any brothers or sisters? Questions tortured me constantly. I didn't know how to stop my mind. What if someone were to find out, or the secret were to spill out of me? Would my life then truly be ruined as I had been led to believe?

I was going through my closet for the third time, trying on skirts, examining and re-examining my body, that I got the idea. I'd get a job. For as long as I could remember, everyone assumed I'd go to college. But that was then. I was no stranger to the world of work. I'd always had a summer job; actually, I'd worked for the government during high school. For the first time since I'd come home, I felt a plan beginning to take form.

Although I was a good student, I'd never won any awards or prizes for anything I'd done in school. I did, however, excel in one thing: typing. I loved to feel my fingers fly over the keyboard of the Smith Corona typewriters that lined the classroom of my high school. My hands took on a life of their own and I entered into a zone that felt almost mystical. When a flyer appeared one day during my sophomore year, announcing that someone was coming to the high school to give civil service exams, my already well-developed fantasy went into overdrive. I wanted desperately to work for the government, make my own money and be independent. Typing was a ticket to the independence I longed for. When calluses appeared on the tips of my fingers from practicing so hard, I paid no attention. The faster I typed, the faster I'd be able to make enough money to do anything I wanted.

I passed the test with flying colors, and spent the summers during high school living out my dream. I was hired as a temporary clerk-typist at the State Department. I loved getting dressed up in stockings and high heels and going to work every day. I had been assigned to work in a typing pool with other girls, all of them much older than I, for the office that specialized in South American affairs. I copied memos from long yellow tablets written by junior staff people who shuffled papers for the embassies throughout South America. I typed names of places like Caracas, Venezuela, and Montevideo, Uruguay; Ecuador; Paraguay—locations that conjured up exotic images of sun-drenched beaches and dark-eyed beauties. The work had little meaning to me and I spent most of my time trying to learn how to operate a copying machine that left my hands stained with blue ink. And yet it was the most adult I had ever felt, and I loved it. The older girls asked me to have lunch with them, and I would sit quietly drinking in their stories of dates and marriages, all the time knowing that it would be a while before I would have that kind of life myself.

After I returned home from Ninny's, I applied for a full-time job back in the State Department. It seemed like a no-brainer and a safe place to land while I figured out my next step. So, when I made the call to Joanne Harrison in the personnel office, it never occurred to me that there would be a problem. It wasn't that we were really friends, but Joanne had treated me well during the time I worked there. She had been in charge of the summer hires that year and had made a point to make me feel at home and not treat me like a kid. I remembered her huge smile and warm voice. I was thrilled when I found out she was still there.

"We'd love to have you back again, Patti," she said on the phone. "I figured you'd be on your way to college by now. I'm surprised you want to apply for a full-time position, but it shouldn't be hard to find you something. Let me call you back in a week or so to set up a meeting to see where you would best fit in." I returned home, confident that I would begin work within a few weeks.

It wasn't until a week before Christmas—five weeks and three days after my conversation with Joanne—that the personnel office finally got back to me. I'd been eagerly counting the days, but every time I called to ask what the hold-up was, I was told to be patient. I couldn't understand why Joanne was taking so long. I reasoned that everyone was probably busy so close to Christmas. When the call did come in, I was a little surprised to hear a voice other than Joanne's. But still, I thought the interview would be a piece of cake. I'd already spent much of the last year waiting and I was more than a little anxious to get on with my life.

I zipped up the new blue wool dress that I had bought for the occasion and slipped into a pair of black high-heeled shoes. It felt good to be in regular clothes again. Although my body had snapped back into shape during the first month after I returned home from the hospital, my breasts had remained larger than before. I ran my hands over my new curves and hoped that Joanne wouldn't notice too much. Little chance, though, as I hadn't seen her in over a year and a half. She would probably think that I had just put on a few pounds and grown up a bit. Maybe it would even help me to get a more interesting job than the typing pool.

Beyond the window of the bus, I could see the sweeping lawns and large colonial houses that lined 16th Street in Washington, D.C. The bus stopped in front of Walter Reed Hospital, where we picked up a couple of passengers, a woman tugging at the hand of a small child bundled in a pink snow-suit and an elderly gentleman wearing a long, navy overcoat and a red scarf, carrying a brief case. It felt good to be back on the familiar bus where, if I close my eyes, I could pretend it was the summer before last, before everything happened, and the only secret I had were the green shoulder pads I used to tuck inside my bra. That sure seemed like a long time ago. With any luck I could begin working by the first of the year. Maybe even sooner.

With shoulders hunched against the wind, I pulled my scarf around my ears and walked the two blocks to Virginia Avenue, where the entrance to the impressive government building was located. It felt good to know where I was going as I pressed the button for the third floor, where the Personnel Office was located. The receptionist, a pretty blonde who didn't look much older than I, waved me to a chair and told me someone would be with me shortly. I peeked around her cubicle to see if I could catch sight of Joanne; but nobody looked familiar, so I sat down to wait. I was glad I'd made this decision. At last everything was falling into place. We'd set up the meeting for three o'clock—five minutes from now. I considered checking myself out in the ladies' room but decided against it, in case Joanne were to appear. I could use a friendly face and really didn't want to miss her. When the door swung open and revealed her, I felt a surge of relief. She glanced at me with a nervous smile, but something was definitely different than I remembered. Joanne was someone you wanted to have lunch with, always made me felt a bit special. This time her voice sounded strangely efficient and terse.

"Your interview will be up on the fifth floor, Patti," she offered, never looking directly at me. "There are a few questions Mr. Donnelly would like to ask. Follow me." There were no words of encouragement, or even polite conversation in the elevator—only awkward silence.

The office was a single room stripped to the essentials: a long library-like table with six wooden chairs lining each side and one at the head. The only suggestion of decoration on the blank white walls was a formal photograph of President Eisenhower that hung on the wall facing the head of the table, and a round clock framed in black. It was ten minutes after three. Joanne introduced me to each of the four men, who I had never seen before, who were seated at the table before making her exit. Suddenly I felt shaky and overwhelmed. One of the men told me to have a seat and pointed to the empty chair at the head of the table. I heard the flicking of a cigarette lighter. Another man carefully placed a pack of Lucky Strike cigarettes on the table and shuffled some papers in front of him.

"We have a few questions we have to ask you, Patti," he said. I straightened my spine and attempted a smile.

"Of course," I said to the ceiling.

Good Girls Don't

The man speaking was probably in his fifties. His hair was receding, almost bald, and he wore a dark suit with a rumpled white shirt and a skinny black tie. He kept reaching for his tie as though to assure himself it was still there,

Another flick of a cigarette lighter; the sound of someone inhaling. "We've gone over your application and it brought up some questions regarding the past year," he said as he blew smoke into the air.

I felt the blood rush to my face, felt the others watching me. "We see you worked at the Pan-American office while you were still in high school. Is that correct?

"Yes, sir," I mumbled. I noticed the fingers of my hand opening and closing as though they belonged to someone else.

"Ordinarily, Patti, this would be just a simple matter of placing you back into the typing pool. We sure could use good typists like you, but there appears to be an irregularity in your application that we feel compelled to explore." He cleared his throat and looked down at the paper in front of him.

Another voice, from the younger man seated across the table from him, took over. "Did you attend business school in McKeesport, Pennsylvania, during the past year?"

If I answered him I might start to cry. Instead I shifted in my seat and studied the area where the paint was peeling off the ceiling. I nodded. "Yes Sir," I replied, barely audible.

"Did you use another name, other than Hawn? Did you use the name Steinhoff?"

I nodded.

"Did you live on Oxford Drive in McKeesport, Pennsylvania, during this time?

I nodded again. Closed my eyes.

'"There appears to be a period of time unaccounted for in your application. Any full-time job with the State Department requires a security clearance. It's a tried-and-true policy legislated by law. This irregularity on your application is serious."

Then, another voice: "We have reason to believe you gave birth to a child out of wedlock, in Washington, D.C. Is this accurate?"

I held my hand up for them to stop, as though I could ward off their questions. I lurched forward and felt as though I was going to throw up.

"We're so terribly sorry, Patti," the bald man added. "As much as we would like to offer you this position, we can't. You would not be able to pass a security clearance."

I rose from my chair, trying to hold back the flood of tears that were waiting to burst, but couldn't stop. I stood there in front of these men and sobbed like a child. The bald man wearing the skinny black tie got up and walked over to me. He put his arm awkwardly around my shoulder and dabbed at my eyes with a crumpled-up handkerchief that he pulled from his pocket.

"I'm so sorry, dear," he said. "This will never leave this room. I wish it could be different."

My shame was complete. I had received the United States government seal of disapproval.

Good Girls Don't

PART II

Found

CHAPTER 18

FROM THE MOMENT I RETURNED HOME from the hospital, my life had been defined by the secret of my pregnancy—my mantle, which I wore like a hair shirt. Although I was a woman with a scarlet past, I had never officially had sex, so I felt like a fraud. And, I was determined—no, obsessed—with changing that status as soon as possible. I felt suspended in time by an unfinished adolescence and a yearning to be an adult. I didn't easily fit into either one of these categories, but I knew that getting a job was a crucial step to becoming an adult and ultimately achieving my independence.

Once again, it was my typing skills, the one thing that never seemed to let me down, that came to my rescue. After my dramatic rejection from the State Department, I found a job working for the National Institutes of Health. No security clearance was asked of me there, and I spent my days typing reports for doctors. Although things were easing up a bit at home, I felt an unspoken sense of disappointment from both of my parents. I was not supposed to be having this life. I should have been graduating from the university and sporting an engagement ring by now. Possibly, if the baby had not been so taboo, and we had talked about the experience, we all might have found a way to allow it to gracefully fade into memory. But the pain stayed stubbornly on the surface, very much alive for all of us.

I was slowly finding my way into the adult world of work and settling into a new routine. I'd met a new friend, Kay, who picked me up at the end of my street each morning and delivered me back in the evening. No one was more surprised than I when one day during our car trip she invited me to go to a dance with her at the Marine base in Quantico, Virginia. "You'll love it," she said. "There are so many cute guys just waiting to meet us. C'mon, Patti, I'll drive. You've got to get out and circulate if you ever want to meet someone." Although the idea sounded a little dangerous, I decided to go. It was fun to feel excited about something again.

It was at that dance that I met Erik Donovan. He was a marine, Irish Catholic and married (which I did not learn until later) --- everything my mother despised, which made him exceedingly attractive.

He was tall, over six feet, with brownish curly hair and a sprinkling of golden freckles across his face. His eyes almost seemed to laugh out loud when he talked, which he did a lot. And he acted as though he had discovered something rare in me, something no one else had ever seen. He told me several times that I was beautiful. What else could I possibly need to know about him?

After the dance at Quantico, Erik and I met for a couple of weeks after work at a smoky jazz club called The Brass Rail where we drank whisky sours and listened to a sultry singer who played great piano. He did most of the talking, about how much he wanted to get out of the Marine Corps. He was from Boston and wanted to get back there as soon as possible. He said he worked for the base newspaper. I assumed he wrote for it, but I never actually was sure. One night I suggested he drive me home. My parents were away, off to the Pocono Mountains for the weekend. Daddy was playing for a group of Saudis who were visiting dignitaries, and Mom had gone along because it was free.

The night was chilly and crisp. When Erik stopped the car in our driveway, he skillfully pressed his hands over my body in an act of ownership that I found both thrilling and dangerous. I didn't hesitate in leaning my body into his. Aren't beautiful women supposed to have sex? We walked into the empty house and I squinted into the bright overhead light. From the front hallway, through the kitchen, I had a view of the back room. I kicked off my high-heeled shoes and walked in my stocking feet toward the large paneled room. The first thing that caught my eye was the photograph of Mom that sat on the mantelpiece where it had always been. Her dark eyes followed me clear across the short walk into the room, making me feel dizzy. My knees shook a little as I removed the photo from the spot, turning her face to the wall. When I turned to look at Erik, I was surprised at how out of place he looked in our back room—like an oversized piece of used furniture that didn't fit. He looked confused for a moment.

"Why did you do that? Is that your mother? I can see where you get your looks," he said, not waiting for an answer. Of course there is not the slightest resemblance between us, but I chose to take it as a compliment anyway. He led me to the worn corduroy chair—the one daddy always sat in to watch television—and pulled me onto his lap.

"Relax, baby, nothing to be nervous about. It's just you and me here and we don't have to rush anything you don't want," he said softly, stroking my hair. "We have all night." I settled into his lap, laying my head against his chest. It felt warm, safe.

"You remind me of a fluffy kitten," he said "From now on I think I'll call you 'Fluffy.' It fits you."

I loved my new nickname; nobody had ever called me anything but Patti.

"I guess I am a little nervous," I confessed. "I've never done this before."

Good Girls Don't

"You mean you're a virgin?" he said, surprised, making it sound almost as though he were ridiculing me.

"I have something to tell you," I began, slowly, cautiously. "I know you're going to find this hard to believe, but, yes, I guess technically I am a virgin." I paused, waiting for this magnificent piece of information to sink in. After all, this was the most important thing about me, actually my entire identity, and I hung on to it with everything I had. I couldn't see his face but I instinctively waited for a sign, a shift in his body, or catch in his breath, something to acknowledge my confession. When I received none of this, not even a reply, I began to feel unsure of myself — but continued my story anyway, attempting a bit more momentum.

"I had a baby last year and I gave him up for adoption. And he, the guy, never even penetrated me." There it was, ragged and raw, dumped stark naked in the middle of the back room, like a huge rotten tomato. "I got pregnant anyway. They, the doctor and everybody, said I was a textbook case. It hardly ever happens to anyone. They removed my whole ovary — told me it was the size of a grapefruit. But that doesn't mean I can't have more kids. Left me with an ugly scar, though. It's fat and runs all the way across my belly. I just thought you should know."

"Must have been awful for you," he said gently. "Don't worry, I know what to do so you won't have anything like that happen to you again. Trust me."

I led Erik up the stairs to my bedroom. My single maple bed, the one with Robert's initials etched in the back of the headboard, startled me in the moment before we switched off the ceiling light and began the business of making love. I wondered when he would bring out the condom, and whether it would be awkward. The desire that had overtaken me earlier in the car had by this time disappeared. After my confession I felt mostly tired, but curiosity more than anything else led me into what happened next.

We removed our clothing in the dark and I quickly slipped under the crisp sheets that Mom always made sure were on my bed. I lay perfectly still on my back, and felt surprise when the unannounced weight of Erik's body landed on top of me. The next thing I knew, he had entered me and my head was banging against the headboard. The rest of my body didn't move much.

All Erik said was that I shouldn't worry because he knew exactly when to pull out. He mumbled something about "being a Catholic and not believing in birth control." It was over before I felt much of anything, except a sore head. When he finished he fell off of me, his arm uncomfortably resting across my breasts, and within a few minutes, maybe seconds, began snoring loudly. I lay there beside him, waiting for the room to stop spinning, and gently pushed his sprawling body as far away from me as I could. It still didn't occur to me to question why on earth I trusted him.

It was after that night in my bedroom that I decided to love him. Sex with Erik might not have been what I thought it should be, but nevertheless I had allowed it to occur, and therefore I needed to sanction it with love. It was as simple as that. And he went happily along with this myth. We saw each other on weekends, usually meeting at The Brass Rail or little restaurants around Dupont Circle in downtown Washington. One time after I told my parents I was spending the night with my new friend from work, we went to a motel, where he assured me that he loved me and wanted to marry me.

This time I knew right away. My breasts, which had not had time to return to their previous size, had become even larger, almost overnight. It was a cold November morning when I pulled

Good Girls Don't

myself out of bed to begin dressing for work. I had just yanked a fuzzy blue cardigan from my dresser when the nausea first drove me into the bathroom. I threw up bile into the toilet and then buried my face into the damp towel that hung over the bathtub and was filled with Daddy's smell. It overtook me, and the violent churning began in my stomach for a second time. This can't be happening to me. Not again. Please God, not again. With difficulty I stumbled back into my bedroom and quietly closed my door, as if by doing so, I could hide from it.

I bundled up against the frigid early morning and walked out into the still, icy air. My throat felt dry as I tied the woolen scarf tightly around my neck. I wandered through the familiar streets of my neighborhood, stopping at a small concrete bridge that crossed high over the railroad tracks near my home. I had always walked quickly over this bridge where Mom had warned me, as a child, never to linger. Many times she had told me the story of our elderly neighbor, Mrs. Gregory, who years ago had lost a child here. For as long as I could remember, the old lady had sat in her upstairs window in a rocking chair surveying the neighborhood, rarely coming out of her house. According to Mom, the mangled body of her seven-year-old boy had been discovered after he had wandered down to this place and fallen to the railroad tracks below. I felt as though I had slipped into a hole in the ground, where I was held hostage inside the possibility of my life as it might have been — and as it would now be.

Fragments of memories from the past year wandered in slow motion across my jagged thoughts. I shuddered — not from the cold, I realized, but because I was sobbing. I leaned forward over the bridge railing and remembered the tears that had streaked Daddy's face after Mom told him of my pregnancy. I don't know how long I remained staring down at the tracks. Finally, it was the vision of the remnants of a blue baby blanket floating across the tops of the trees, bending under the wind that pulled me away from the frightening comfort I 'found in the abyss. I furiously lurched myself away and began running back home.

Mom was sitting in the back room sipping a cup of coffee when I returned. "You're up early," she said, her eyes peering at me like she was waiting for bad news. "What got you out of bed so early on a Saturday morning?"

I would sooner have died than to utter the words that I knew I must. That once again I had disappointed her. "I'm pretty sure I'm pregnant again, Mom. I'm so sorry to put you through all of this -- after everything…..", my voice was calmer than I thought possible. "I'm so, so sorry…Mom just sighed. I braced myself for what would come next, but nothing else followed. The sigh had said it all. Her spirit—usual willingness to jump into the moment, as was her way, had for now left her. Her face crumpled under the weight of the sigh taking on the texture of crinkled tissue paper.

"I'm going to marry Erik, Mom—nothing else matters. Don't worry about me, I'll handle this.

I spent the first few days after I knew for sure that I was pregnant in an unconscious haze.

I was sure of one thing without a doubt: that I would never under any circumstances give this baby away. In the days and weeks that followed it was this resolve that led me down the difficult path of Erik Donovan's life.

I called Erik at the base the following day. I'd been holding the phone for almost ten minutes, waiting for Erik to be located at the base before finally, they found him in the barracks.

Good Girls Don't

"I need to see you right away. It's an emergency."

"Hold on baby, what's wrong?"

"Erik, I'm pregnant. I know it. I'm sick, I just know. I'm going to have a baby. Oh my God, Erik, what am I going to do?"

He didn't miss a beat. His voice—silky smooth—never changed.

"Nothing to worry about, Fluffy. We'll get married, just as soon as I can make some arrangements."

These are the words I hung onto during the next couple of weeks, until I saw him next.

The nights were the worst. In the daylight I could pretend that we loved each other and we'd be married, but alone in my bed, in the middle of the night, the truth seeped through. Erik didn't love me, and for that matter, I didn't love him. During one of those nights I bolted out of bed, careful not to wake my parents, and descended into the basement. The stairs groaned under my weight. I turned on the light bulb that hung from the ceiling of the cold cellar, strangely unfamiliar in the middle of the night. I pulled the towel around me from the clothesline that extended across the room, fumbling in the eerie light until I found a cardboard box hidden behind Daddy's watch-repair books. This is the box that Erik had asked me, a couple of weeks ago, to keep for him, saying he needed more space than the locker in his barracks would allow. I sat on the bottom step and ripped through the heavy masking tape that sealed it. I supposed that Erik thought because the box was sealed it was safe from my discovering it's contents. Or, possibly, he may have secretly wanted me to know the truth but didn't have the courage to tell me. Sitting on top was a photograph of Erik standing beside a tall blonde girl under a palm tree. The sun blurred her face so I couldn't see much of what she looked like. It was his hand that caught my attention. It reached easily around her slender waist, touching her stomach as though he was patting it—a gesture so intimate I had to look away. I hurried on to the next layer of papers: a high school diploma, an official envelope from the Marine Corps—and then, tucked underneath some blank post cards, the letters, six of them. The envelopes were addressed to someone named Kate Donovan, postmarked two years before. They looked as if they had been returned unopened. I tore open the first envelope, almost as though I already knew the contents, and there I learned the astounding fact that Erik was already married to a woman named Kate, who lived in Miami, with their two-year-old little girl, Debbie. Only after reading the letter that began "Dear Fluffy" did I stop long enough to gasp for air. Momentarily dizzy, I closed my eyes so tightly that little flashes of light streaked across my eyelids, eventually melting into a single image: the face of my baby boy, his eyes locking into mine.

Eventually I stood up, stumbled across the room and mounted the creaking stairs. I kept asking myself, what am I going to do? But by the time the pale morning light filled the back room, and my tears had dried up. I knew. I realized that nothing this man had told me about himself was true—and, perversely, this brought me a strange sense of freedom. It somehow strengthened my commitment to get what I needed: his name. There was no shame too deep or humiliation too humbling for me to stop until I got it.

After that night, I became a calculating machine with the single-minded purpose of finding refuge in the only societal endorsement that could possibly protect me and my unborn child: marriage. In my mind, it was the only power that could legitimize, actually condone, our existence. Nothing else mattered. I even concocted the idea that Kate must want to divorce Erik. Why else would they be apart? But I needed to know for sure. Without hesitating, I found her phone number from Miami information. It did not register as bold or even unusual for me to make the call. It was simply the next step

Good Girls Don't

Kate answered the phone on the first ring, almost as if she had been waiting to hear from me. I spilled out my story without taking a breath and then waited for what seemed an eternity for her reply. Her voice was slow, soft, distinctly southern, each word standing alone.

"That lousy son-of-a-bitch bastard did it again. Sugar, we're going to nail that no-good mother fucker. You just hang on, I'm flying up there tomorrow and we'll get his Irish ass. You can write your name on that."

I let out a sigh and told her all I cared about was getting Erik to marry me, no matter what that took. After that, I'd get a divorce, never see him again I didn't care. We talked for over an hour. She told me her story: she'd met him a few years ago when he was stationed in Miami; she'd married him to get away from home, and soon realized it was a big mistake after she got pregnant and caught him lying about everything.

"That guy even lied about stuff that would have served him better to tell the truth. Like he couldn't help it, or something."

Mom had oddly become a partner to my plan of finding a way to marry Erik Donovan. She readily invited Kate to stay at our home during this charade. I guess she knew this young woman held the key to the legitimacy of her grandchild, and she was not going to leave any stoned unturned, no matter how distasteful, to assure this eventuality. She was not going to lose another grandchild. It was actually her idea for the two of us to drive to the base the next night, and Kate quickly agreed.

The next night I climbed out of a cab at National Airport, and headed immediately to the ladies' room, where I checked myself out in the harsh overhead light. Yanking a comb through my tangled hair, I stared at my face — puffy, pale, with dark circles under my eyes. I patted a little pancake make-up under them but only made it worse. I wanted desperately to make a good impression on

Kate. After all, she was coming all this way to…I'm not exactly sure what she was going to do, but at this moment, she was my lifeline.

I checked and discovered that the plane was on time. It was almost midnight and I was exhausted, but this was the flight Kate had chosen, and for sure I wasn't going to disappoint her. I watched as the passengers filed past the arrival gate, peering into each face, until I heard a soft drawl inquire, "Are you Patti?"

The voice belonged to a stunning, tall blonde who looked to me like she just stepped out of the pages of a fashion magazine. Her hair was swept up in a glamorous French twist that accentuated her long gracious neck. She was wearing high-heeled shoes and a fitted gray suit and her lips were outlined with a shade of raspberry that I'd never seen.

"Yes," I stammered. "I'm Patti. Thank you so much for doing this. I didn't really know where to turn. Thank you." My voice trailed off. I never expected anyone this glamorous. All I could think of to do was grab her small overnight case, which she immediately took from my hand.

"Give me that," she said, grabbing the case. "You have enough to carry right there."

She patted my belly like we were old friends, and then she looked at me for a long time, her pale blue eyes hinting at an unspoken secret between us. For a moment I almost believed everything was going to work out.

I never had a conversation with Daddy about my pregnancy, but of course he knew. Mom told him. He spent more time taking naps behind the closed bedroom door, never confronting me, but always appearing to be clothed in a veil of shadowy sadness. Mom, on the other hand, became a partner to my plan of finding a way to marry Erik. This young woman held the key to the legitimacy of her grandchild, and she was not going to leave any stoned unturned, no matter how distasteful, to assure this eventuality. It was Mom's idea for the two of us to drive to the base the next night, and I quickly agreed.

"We'll catch him right as he's leaving work," Kate said. "He'll be completely off guard, never know what hit him. I can't wait to see his face."

She made plans, rehearsed dialogue, and then changed it, added twists. By the time we began the drive to Quantico, her mood was almost feverish, just short of ecstatic at the prospect of cornering him. It had begun to occur to me that this was far less about me than it was about her getting back at Erik. I had to keep reminding myself that Kate had flown up here from Miami to help me and for this I would always be grateful. I was growing a little confused, however, about what her motives for the trip really were. I buried these feelings as we began the drive to the marine base. I reminded myself that I had only one goal and needed to remain single minded to this. I was somehow going to marry this man and keep this baby. That's as far ahead as I could plan.

"He's going to pee his pants when he sees me with you," she said gleefully. "I'd like to bottle the look on his face. Can't wait, can you?"

I nodded, nervously. Without argument I agreed to every hair-brained idea, no matter how self-serving or foolish, that she hurled at me. I hadn't added anything to the conversation for miles. Like a sawdust puppet, I sat there, an accomplice to something — I just didn't know what. All I wanted was for her to sign a divorce paper, which, I'd learned, she'd held onto for the last couple of years because she was afraid she'd lose the allotment she received from the Marine Corps as his wife. She told me that she had met someone else and had been ready for a divorce for over a year but just hadn't gotten around to it. Her marriage to Erik was a sham and she, too, had been duped initially by his charm.

"He calls me all the time," she continued. "Always wants to get back with me, acts like he cares about Debbie, but he's only seen her once." None of this surprised me somehow, but what she said next did: "He was in Miami just a few weeks ago, begged us to come back, said he'd take care of us this time."

"You mean you saw him in Miami?" I was incredulous.

"Yeah. I guess he was trying to get out of his latest mess…with you, I mean."

A mess. I guess I am a mess, I thought barely out of my teens, sitting in a car with this woman who I barely knew, pregnant and unmarried for the second time in two years. I was definitely on the verge of losing my nerve by the time we arrived at the base. Kate seemed to know exactly where to find him. By this time I had stopped questioning anything about her, figured I'd find out everything sooner or later.

When I first saw Erik he was standing outside the entrance to a one-story building that looked like a stationary trailer. Kate, who had endlessly choreographed exactly where we would stand to provide the most dramatic impact, was positively bubbling with excitement. I saw him before he saw us and heroically fought the urge to look away as he began to walk toward us. His eyes widened, but only briefly, as he approached. If he was shocked, it was barely visible. There was a brief flicker of recognition as his eyes moved over my face but not a hint of surprise.

He looked right through me to Kate, and said without hesitation. "I don't know what she's told you. But that baby probably isn't even mine. She had one and gave it up for adoption last year. Who knows who she's been with."

I answered him with silence but noticed a rigid set to Kate's jaw after he spoke. She waved me into the car, where I stayed for

Good Girls Don't

what seemed like hours while they went somewhere to talk privately. When they returned, holding hands, Kate spoke first.

"It's all settled. I will go back to Miami and begin divorce proceedings. You marry him and after the baby is born, you get a divorce. That way everybody gets what they want. Right, honey?" She tilted her beautiful face up at him and smiled. "And then, Erik and I can probably get back together again. Only this time, we'll do it right."

Erik simply nodded to whatever she said, agreeing to this outlandish idea, mumbling that "it's obviously the right thing to do."

It was only after we got back into the car to return to my home that Kate told me she had "no intention of ever letting that sorry piece of Irish ass" back into her life. "Not ever! We girls have to stick together; it's all we really have," she added.

Sometime during that night, inside the freezing car, I rid myself of any illusions I ever had about love, or for that matter, marriage—an erasure that held for some thirty years. A hole opened up inside my heart and swallowed Erik and Kate so completely that when they returned to the car to tell me that they had agreed to a divorce, it was as though amnesia had taken over and for many years, I barely had any recollection of the event. Sometimes if I walked into a musty room, or heard a version of Mendelssohn's *Wedding March*, a dim stab of pain would carry me back to an incomplete remnant of that day

---

The house, somewhere in Arlington, Virginia, had a small sign, "Justice of the Peace," tacked onto the front door. Even though it was the middle of the afternoon, the tiny living room was dark and stifling hot, like an attic filled with unwanted dusty pillows and flowers left too long in their vases. The sweet smell of overripe bananas, left in a bowl on the table, overcame me and I was sure I'd gag. The judge's eyes were buried in deep wrinkles that lined every inch of his face. He asked us to stand in front of the bananas and repeat after him. A woman with fat jowls that reached past her chin appeared out of nowhere, and the old man commanded her to stand beside me. She was the witness, my maid of honor. He began speaking, stopped, and abruptly reached behind some magazines on a shelf. He found a phonograph record with no cover. Soon a scratchy version of Jo Stafford singing *The Wedding March* filled the room.

The next thing I remembered was the fat lady bringing me a jelly glass filled with water. I had apparently fainted.

My son, Michael was born two weeks later. He was a beautiful baby boy with bright red hair like mine, and shocking blue eyes that looked as though they were laughing out loud.

I divorced Erik one month after Michael was born.

CHAPTER 19

AFTER MICHAEL'S BIRTH I was taken over by a new and unfamiliar feeling. I thought of myself no longer as an individual, but as part of an inseparable duo. It was the early sixties, and there were few role models for single moms, so I was swimming in uncharted waters. If I thought I needed a husband before his birth, my son provided me with a restless drive to find him a father.

When Michael was two months old I returned to my job at the National Institutes of Health; a month later I moved out of my parents' home. My salary barely covered my living expenses. My one-bedroom walk-up apartment on the third floor in a suburban area of Silver Spring cost $77 a month and the baby-sitter was another fifty dollars.

Every morning I woke up Michael at exactly 6 a.m. and fed him a bottle that had been prepared the night before. I had learned to prop the bottle on a folded blanket and place him on his side so he could drink it while I was getting dressed for work. I knew he'd rather have me hold him, but there was no time. I had 30 minutes to get dressed, make my tea and toast, which I ate in the car, and drive him to the baby-sitter — a neighbor who lived down the street from my parents. I slipped into my high heels, placed Michael over my shoulder and began my climb down the three flights of stairs and into the car for the fifteen-minute drive. Leah, the sitter, would be waiting at her front door for me to silently place my baby into her arms.

This ritual was repeated each day for several weeks until Mom made a surprise visit to Leah's house one afternoon and found Michael crying in his makeshift crib. She decided that the arrangement was unsuitable and he was not getting proper care. She told me that from now on she would be taking care of him, and I could give her the $50 a month. I agreed. She loved Michael dearly, and although there were times when he became a bargaining chip between us, I knew he would receive the best possible care.

My decision to move into my own apartment had been an obvious declaration of my desire for independence, but I wasn't prepared for the realities of living alone with an infant. Mom may have disapproved of practically everything about my life, but she was by no means going to give up the care of her grandson. I might have moved into a new physical space, but I was still tightly tethered to my family. And Michael was the bond that kept that tie securely knotted.

With money so tight, I thought it would help to have a roommate, so I placed an ad in the Washington Post: Single mother wishes to share one-bedroom apartment with same. Please call between the hours of 6 and 9 pm. The first night the ad appeared I received 17 calls from women ranging from very young to middle aged, and they all shared one thing: they sounded desperate. Marianne Morley moved in with me within a day of answering my ad. While hers was definitely not the most desperate-sounding call, she clearly was needy enough to move into an apartment with only one double bed. Marianne had a six-month-old boy named Ricky. Although we never discussed his father or much about her past, we did talk about options for our sleeping arrangements.

This included an extremely uncomfortable early-American style wooden couch that Ninny had given me. During our first cup of tea together, we decided, due to our limited funds, to share the double bed, at least until Marianne could save enough from her government salary to buy her own bed. We put Ricky's crib in an alcove off the kitchen known as a dinette.

"You're what?" Mom shrieked when she heard of my plan. "Who is this girl? Have you completely lost your mind? Don't you understand that you have a child now — and that has to come before anything else? You are obviously not capable of taking care of yourself, much less a child." She was cradling Michael in her arms while saying this, holding him to her as though protecting him from me.

"He is mine," I screamed at her, surprised at this new, unfamiliar voice. "He doesn't belong to you. I'm his mother, not you."

I was across the room in one leap and in a blind rage tried to pull Michael from her arms. She held on to him even tighter.

By the time Daddy walked into the room, we were in the midst of a tug-of-war with Michael as the prize, both screaming at the top of our voices. Daddy never uttered a word, but took the baby away from Mom and walked out of the room, carrying him upstairs. By this time I was hysterical, screaming at the top of my lungs that I hated her. I never saw her hand as it flew across my face. I froze with shock; for a split second I considered running, but instantly knew the futility of this and simply waited, trembling and speechless. Finally, the years of pain and disappointment were exposed between us, and my mother's face reflected the fear she must have felt about everything that lay ahead for me. Every dream she had for my life had been shattered. Since she had never learned how to differentiate between her own life and that of her children, it must have been extraordinarily difficult for her to feel so helpless, watching me slip away from her protective cloak.

Nothing really changed after that incident. Mom and I never apologized to each other, or for that matter ever discussed our relationship in any depth. Although her disapproval of my life never waivered, she continued, for the next few years, to take care of Michael during the day while I worked. Apparently we both needed each other for our own reasons and continued to play out this elaborate game that included my desire to prove, at all costs, that she was wrong—and hers to continue to prove she was the better parent to my son.

As I began to make more money, Marianne and I eventually moved into a two- bedroom apartment in a slightly more upscale development. I typed my way through the next several years, moving easily from one job to the next. When I moved out of the typing pool and began working for a lobbyist at the Motion Picture Association in Washington, I also worked nights for a law firm a few blocks away. When I was asked to spend a month working for a congressman at the Capitol, I led everyone to believe I could take shorthand, a requirement for the job. I would often spend hours after Michael was in bed transcribing my scribbled notes so that I could read them to type up the following day.

When my car broke down on the way home from work one evening, I pulled into a gas station where I saw an old Pontiac with a big white stripe painted around its chassis and a for-sale sign propped on the windshield. I bought it on the spot for 200 dollars. No matter that it was an unfamiliar stick shift: I learned how to drive it on the way home.

In the early 1960's, Washington was ripe with the youthful hope of the Kennedy administration, and the city was infused with the energy of attractive young government workers, all trying to make their mark. My office was located a few blocks from the White House, so I could watch the planes take off from Andrews Air force Base during the Cuban Missile Crisis. Although most of Washington spent those days with transistor radios held against their ears, I was far too absorbed in taking care of my own life to muster much fear. When I went to pick Michael up one evening during this time, Mom tersely handed me a ten-dollar bill and told me to stash it in my glove compartment. "You never have enough gas," she said. "I don't want you to be stranded if the city needs to evacuate." She then handed me some cans of peaches and corn to carry to the basement "in the event of an attack." (If my practical mother was stashing canned goods in the basement, it got my attention).

There was no lack of party invitations and young men to date during these years, and there was only one strict rule: my dates had to agree up front to pay my baby-sitter. Mom had no problem taking care of Michael while I worked, but she had no intention of supporting my social life.

One Saturday night I went with a couple of girlfriends from my office to a party in Arlington, Virginia. All we knew was that it was being hosted by a group of young, single lawyers from the Justice Department. That seemed like a good enough reason to show up. The front door was ajar, and we could hear the sounds of the Supremes floating toward us as we got off the elevator. All I could see through the smoke-filled living room was a haze of wall-to-wall people: sleek-looking office girls in little black dresses that skimmed their bodies, and men in three-button suits and slim dark ties, a few of whom had already begun to let their hair grow longer.

I pulled out a compact from my purse, re-applied my lipstick, and tucked the ends of my hair into the new French twist that I'd recently begun wearing. I reached for a cigarette from a tray on the coffee table, but before I could find a match, a stunning man appeared holding a lighter. "Hey, my name is Gregg. Actually, Gregory, but everyone calls me Gregg. Can I get you a drink?" he said.

"Thanks, " I answered. "I'll have a scotch and water." I had only begun trying this drink because I'd been told it would be less likely to make me sick than cocktails with sugar mixes. I didn't much like how it tasted but I liked ordering it. It sounded more sophisticated to me. When he went to fetch my drink I had a chance to notice that he was at least six feet tall, with a strong, athletic-looking body, short-cropped blond hair, and a chiseled face that set off clear blue eyes. He handed me the drink with such force that it crashed into my arm, spilling all over my dress, and when he grabbed a tiny cocktail napkin and clumsily patted my arm with it, he spilled even more of if down the front of my dress. I didn't get mad, though. There was something endearing about his clumsiness that actually made me want to comfort him.

"I'm so sorry," he said earnestly. "I'm really sorry. Hope I didn't ruin your dress." As he furiously continued to pat me down I began to laugh. He told me he had been going to George Washington University off and on for quite a while. He didn't ask much about me but spoke of arriving in New York with his family when he was twelve. I think he told me he played tennis on a scholarship somewhere, and that he worked on construction jobs to pay for school. Mostly we didn't talk much, but danced. When the Supremes gave way to Frank Sinatra I liked how I fit against his chest. There was something about his bigness that made me feel safe.

Although Gregg and I dated for almost a year, he periodically warned me he was not ready for the responsibility of marriage, and certainly not fatherhood. And I knew this was true. He was a big, overgrown kid — easy to like, but nobody you really wanted to count on. And yet, he was so comfortable and fun to be with that I continued seeing him. One night as we were on our way to the movies he stopped at a deli and filled bags with pastrami sandwiches and sour pickles and sides of potato salad laced with pungent garlic. We hid the bags inside my purse and shared the food inside the theater, giggling together. Gregg remained oblivious as people began to clear a space around us; he continued to chomp on his sandwich, offering me bites of pickles as though we were sitting in a restaurant. He was a man who clearly claimed his space with a flourish. Even if he pissed you off, you couldn't help liking him.

It was impossible not to choose political sides during the spring of 1963, so when Gregg decided to avoid the draft by joining the National Guard, I was completely supportive, even turned on by his decision. As part of his commitment he spent six months at Fort Dix in New Jersey and arrived home on the chilly morning of November 22, 1963. We had spoken the previous night on the phone and had agreed to meet at my friend's apartment where we could be alone. We had seen each other periodically during the six months he was in training, but his absence had definitely worked toward obscuring the realities of Gregg's flaws as a potential husband.

I was taking the day off work and had spent the morning at the apartment preparing for his arrival. I filled the refrigerator with food I knew he liked — fresh fruit, salami, the hearty German bread from the deli. Fiddling with the radio, I found a jazz station that played romantic ballads, and I left the front door cracked open so that I'd be the first thing he saw when he got off the elevator. Finally, I heard the elevator door close, and his large frame filled the doorway. At that point any doubt I may have had about him went flying into a back corner of my brain. He was wearing his uniform and looked like he belonged in a military recruitment ad. All the pent-up need for a husband found its way to my tongue and I blurted out, "I've missed you so much. I don't ever want to be separated from you again."

"Me too," he answered, picking me up in his arms, his voice cracking with emotion. "It's been so lonely without you." He continued, his voice animated, "I've had time to do a lot of thinking and all I know is that I love you."

The radio was playing a Nat King Cole song about summer love when he kissed me—a long, deep kiss that I wanted to last forever, but eventually the song ended and so did the kiss. All of a sudden the radio became louder and a man's voice filled the room.

"The President has been shot," the voice said. "I repeat: President Kennedy has been shot."

The words were incomprehensible, jarring us out of this private moment as if a silent explosion had splattered deep inside of the borrowed apartment. As we untangled our arms, all I remember was the roar of blood in my ears. I grabbed my purse, found my cigarettes and forced smoke into my lungs, the cigarette helping me remember how to breathe.

Gregg and I didn't know what to say to each other, so we were silent. We walked out into the chilly November air together, climbed into my striped blue Pontiac and began mindlessly driving toward downtown. The radio kept feeding us more information, making it real. It seemed we had a mutual pull to be in the heart of the city.

We drove silently through Georgetown and Pennsylvania Avenue, finally ending up in a small Italian restaurant in Foggy Bottom where we knew the owner. Everyone was crowded around the small television set at the bar. A man I'd never seen poured me a glass of beer and then hugged me, and I hugged him back. Later that evening we drove by a church on 16th Street and wordlessly pulled into the parking lot and walked inside, where we joined hands with another group of people—some crying, some praying—and listened to a preacher try to make sense of a world that we all knew would never be the same.

By the end of that day Gregg and I were convinced that together we had moved through something so profound that our relationship had forever changed. "I think we should get married," I said solemnly. Gregg nodded in agreement. It seemed like the only right thing to do.

Michael, who was four years old when I married Gregg, was the best man at our impromptu wedding. We were married by a young rabbi Mom had found for us—Mom, Daddy, Ninny and Uncle Charlie all awkwardly circling us during the ceremony, waiting for Gregg to bolt. After the Kennedy tragedy he had postponed the wedding so many times that Uncle Charlie forgot the new date and almost missed it. Gregg always got scared the night before and would break down crying and tell me he wasn't sure he was ready for the responsibility, but that he loved me and didn't want us to break up. The last time he did this Ninny called him and told him to "either shit or get off the pot," so I guess it was the nudge he needed.

We were an odd wedding party: Mom pretending to hold Gregg up as they got into the car and Michael with a droopy daisy pinned to his little jacket. Daddy even asked me in the car if I was really sure this is what I wanted.

"Look," I answered. "Michael needs a father, and he's a good guy."

Sometimes I wonder if I married him because he was so good looking—big, tall, blonde, with strong chiseled features. I was so envious of all my girlfriends, who by now were married and living in housing developments in the suburbs, that I could think of little else. All I wanted was to live in one of those split-level houses with a family room and a kitchen, where I could make exotic dishes, like beef stroganoff, for small dinner parties.

Above anything else I wanted a Daddy for Michael. I'd been a single mom trying to raise him by myself, and I was frankly tired of it. For some unexplained reason, Gregg seemed to fit into my family fantasy. Behind his loud, boisterous personality I couldn't help but believe he was a good guy. I liked the way he charged into rooms like a brisk wind, reminding me of a big clumsy bull, only good looking. I figured he just hadn't quite grown up yet.

Any deep analysis of my new husband was put off indefinitely when I learned I was pregnant. From the second I discovered I was going to have another baby I slipped inside a bubble that nothing could burst. This time I believed I'd gotten it right. After going through two pregnancies alone, I was finally official, a married lady with a handsome husband. I didn't even care that the split-level house that I longed for had never materialized, or that Gregg couldn't seem to handle money and had gotten us deeply into debt. Everyone else I knew was doing well, moving up and out into larger worlds, or so it seemed, I skimped on everything, but was never able to break even. Gregg was always going back to school to get his business degree, but when it came time to pay the tuition he never had the money. I kept telling myself that he meant well, that he'd grow up, but most of the time I felt as though I was living with a very large child.

One late afternoon, however, I had taken off work to do some last-minute preparations for the coming baby, hoping I could complete a project before Gregg came home from his construction job. I was down in the basement of our small town house putting the finishing touches on a dresser for the baby I'd picked up at a garage sale. I'd painted it bright yellow and was in the midst of replacing the pulls with large alphabet blocks, just like I'd seen in *Good Housekeeping Magazine*, when the phone rang. The voice on the other end sounded startled when I said "hello."

"Does Gregg live here?" asked a giggling young girl. I answered that he did and could hear whispering in the background.

"Who is this?" I asked, but by this time she had hung up.

I put the receiver back into the cradle, but before I could walk away it rang again. This time I answered during the first ring but all I heard was a rude click. I thought it odd but decided to let it go. Gregg was still at the construction site, ironically working on one of those suburban houses I dreamed of, and not due home for another hour or so. I made a mental note to tell him about the strange calls during dinner, but I was far too happy to let anything interfere. No dark thoughts were allowed to come even close. I was about to give birth to my baby, a little brother or sister for Michael, and nothing was going to get in the way of my happiness.

By the time Gregg came home I was still lost in my furniture project and had forgotten about the phone calls, although there had been another hang-up an hour later. I had some big news to tell him tonight. I'd finally decided on the baby's name. Our deal was that if it was a girl he would name it and if it turned out to be a boy it was my choice. I knew it was a boy, never had a moment's doubt.

It was a Tuesday night, in January 1967, and almost immediately after returning home, Gregg, who blew off everything else, was off to his National Guard meeting. During the three years we were married I couldn't remember one Tuesday that he had missed, not ever. When I teased him about his commitment to his country, he would bristle and say that if he didn't go he would probably be drafted and end up in Viet Nam and did I want to be a war widow?

"I've decided on his name." I yelled from the basement when I heard him approach the door. "Do you want to know?"

"No, wait," he answered. "If you're right and it's a boy, you can tell me after he's born. It'll be more of a surprise that way."

I liked his answer. Maybe he's finally getting into this, I thought. He'd been so lukewarm about the baby since he found out I was pregnant. I guessed some guys were like that, though. They needed to hold the baby in their arms before they could feel anything.

I lumbered up the steps to say good-bye to Gregg. I knew he'd be gone in a few minutes and was feeling strangely warm toward him tonight. My due date was two weeks away and I was huge. I'd grown so large during my pregnancy the doctor at first thought I was going to have twins. I grabbed onto the kitchen table for support and reached over to give him a peck on the cheek.

"Don't you want something to eat? There's leftover spaghetti. I'll warm it up."

"No," he answered over his shoulder. "I'll grab something on the way." He stood up and left the room, and in a few minutes, I heard the shower running. When he came back downstairs dressed to go out, he glanced at me standing in the kitchen.

"I may be late, so don't wait up." He grazed my cheek as he passed me and went out the kitchen door to the garage, stopping only for a minute in front of the mirror to smooth his short-cropped hair with his hands. I thought of running out after him to ask about the strange phone calls, but decided against it.

After I put Michael to bed I sat down to watch television but felt bored, a little uncomfortable. I knew Gregg's meeting started promptly at seven and he would have had no time to eat, so I decided to surprise him with an impromptu late-night dinner. It was already close to 11, and I knew he'd be home soon. I pulled out the leftover spaghetti, thought better of it and instead decided on two steaks I'd been saving in the freezer for a special occasion, like after I came home from the hospital. Why wait, I thought. I've decided on the baby's name; that surely deserves a steak. I was too excited to wait as Gregg had suggested, and decided to write the baby-boy name on a card and slip it under his plate. I pulled out the good china that Mom had insisted everyone in the family buy for us but that we'd never used, carefully placed the delicate crystal wine glasses beside the china. I set the table with a creamy linen tablecloth and candles, tossed together a salad and chopped up some fresh chives into a tiny cut-glass bowl of sour cream. I glanced at the clock in the kitchen and was surprised that an entire hour had passed. I guess I'd been pretty lost in my love meal.

As I lit the candles and stood back to admire my beautiful table, I felt something akin to a burst water balloon pour out between my legs. For a moment I thought I'd actually wet my pants, but it only took a second or two to realize my water had broken. Even though I was having no contractions, or at least no pain, by now I knew enough about the process of childbirth to realize that I needed to get off my feet fast. No reason to panic, I thought. This kind of thing happens all the time.

I walked into the bedroom and put on a fresh pair of underwear, changed into a clean maternity skirt and returned to the kitchen where I pulled a chair up to the phone and dialed information. I asked for the number of the National Guard in Silver Spring. It took forever for someone to answer; when they finally did, I asked the sleepy voice on the other end of the phone if the meeting had ended and, if so, what time. I think I included that it was an emergency.

"Sorry, lady, I don't know nothing about any meeting. I'm just here finishing up some paper work. Nobody else here but me."

"No, you don't understand," I continued. "It's Tuesday night. It's the National Guard meeting night. You know, every Tuesday," I repeated. "I've got to find my husband and he's there. Would you please look for him? It's urgent."

"Hey lady, sorry, there's no meeting here. We stopped doing those Guard meetings over five years ago. Somebody's pulling your leg. Are you all right? Do you want me to call someone?"

I replaced the receiver, staring at it in disbelief. I rose and switched off the television, and walked into Michael's room and looked at my little boy, his arms and legs sprawled over the edge of his bed. I leaned over, grabbing my belly, and tucked the blanket around him, then moved back to the dark living room like a sleepwalker. It all crashed through the numb jumble of my mind at once—the phone calls from strangers, the lack of interest in the baby, the lies about car trouble and late night study groups with buddies. He had lied to me about everything. It was just like the other times; I'd have this baby alone, too.

I stood up to call the doctor, but realized that my entire body was shaking. I looked at the steaks sitting on the table waiting to be cooked, the knife lying beside it. I imagined stabbing Gregg through the heart, again and again, when he walked through the door. I was breathing in short gasps, unable to get air into my chest. I began to cry—wild, uncontrollable sobs. I looked at the perfect table and smashed my fists into the dinner plate, watched as it shattered on the floor. The little card I had placed under the dish, with the name "David" scribbled on it and underneath the word "beloved," was all that remained.

I sat on the floor holding the card, rocking back and forth, my hands wrapped around my enormous belly, already beginning to plot my survival.

"Breathe, Patti. You need to keep breathing." The nurse at the hospital held my hand tightly. I think I'm going to die, the pain is so intense. Then, suddenly, it subsides a little and I am able to catch my breath. I look around the hospital room and see Gregg standing at the foot of the bed. I turn my head away from him and instead look at the nurse. I want to block him from my view, from my life. He has no right to be here.

The doctor stands over me and asks if I'm ready for something to help with the pain.

"Sure," I say numbly, "I'll take anything I can get for pain. I'm worn out from it."

Good Girls Don't

I look up to see Gregg avert his eyes from me as they wheel me out into the delivery room.

After David's birth I realized my marriage to Gregg was essentially over, but it took me close to six years to admit it and find the courage to leave. I filled up the spaces in my unhappy marriage working at a crisis intervention agency in Maryland. I worked there for five years, and by the time I left I was chief of everything from talking down the hordes of suburban white kids who were in the midst of bad drug trips, to fighting with the funding agencies to secure housing for chronic alcoholics. It was a clearing-house for all the backlash of the sixties that had sprung up inside the pristine suburban neighborhoods. If there was anything left of my used-up passion, it was lavished on my children and my job. I tried to fill up my own emptiness with the unfortunates of the world, taking on each one of them as though their life depended on me. It was only after I learned that it was my life that depended on them that things really began to fall apart. I guess the divorce was inevitable; at least that's what the army of shrinks I consulted told me. For a time I had my therapist, Gregg had his, and we had ours. These were the primary gurus. They, in turn, each had their legions of counselors, human potential leaders, self-help masters and eastern religious pundits. The array of people selling their brands of life's answers was dazzling. And there were days when I think we visited the majority of them.

During this period of time Mom and I got into the habit of meeting for lunch at a local Chinese restaurant. She was managing a jewelry store that was close to my office, and for an hour each week I would confide my list of bitter marital complaints to her. Although it had been pouring down rain for three days we had agreed to meet, as usual, but by the time I arrived, and spotted her in a corner booth, I was dripping wet and in a foul mood.

"You're soaked to the skin," she began. "Don't you believe in umbrellas?"

I ignored her, and began speaking as though we were in the midst of an ongoing conversation — one that was predictable and had absolutely nothing to do with the moment.

"I don't know, Mom — ever since that National Guard thing, everything's wrong; it never got better. It was a long time ago but I suspect he's probably still screwing around, and the worst is, I don't even care much anymore. Something's wrong if you don't care. You know what I mean? When I married him I thought he was different, so good-looking, those piercing blue eyes, the way he played tennis. I used to love the way his shoulders filled out his shirt."

"Wonderful credentials for marriage," Mom erupted. "Especially the shoulders. Christ, if you'd ever get past the shoulders, possibly look inside the head, you might have a chance."

I paid little attention to her, having grown used to her colorful critiques. It was a tradeoff: I got to complain and she got to criticize, usually me.

"Well at least you're back at work; that's one good thing. At least you're not sitting at home answering phone calls from creditors."

I smoothed my new mini-skirt over my thighs and reached for another portion of fried rice.

"Who knows," I said, completely ignoring her, continuing our mutually independent conversations. "Maybe when the kids are a little older, it'll get easier."

"I've told you again and again, Patti. It never gets easier. It just keeps getting a little worse. You say the first hurtful thing to each other and that's kind of hard but the next time it gets easier, just slips out, and then it's real easy, like falling off a log and you're off and running. Everything always gets just a little bit worse."

She filled my plate with more mu shu pork and poured me another cup of tea.

"Wow, Mom. You're in a particularly inspiring mood today," I said. "Look. We're getting into couples counseling. Pretty crazy, huh? You and Dad ever think about doing that? Never know, might have helped things."

I awaited her next zinger, but surprisingly she was quiet—just sat staring out the window at the rain with the saddest expression I'd ever seen her wear. It's not like we hadn't said this same stuff to each other for years. It was our game, what we did, and what we always expected to do. Only this time, she wasn't playing.

"Mom, I have to get back to work. I'll call you later. Don't worry, I'll figure it out, or not. One way or the other, you know I'm fine."

She continued to stare out the window into the pouring rainstorm as though I'd already left.

"Mom, are you OK? Is something wrong? You're scaring me. Say something. It's your serve."

She pulled her eyes away from the window and looked at me as if I'd just gotten there. She took a pack of menthol cigarettes from her purse and offered me one. Her face was pale.

"Sit down. You're already late for work. I have something to tell you."

I placed the car key in my hand as though ready to put it into the ignition right there at the table. Something in Mom's voice warned me that whatever she was about to say, I didn't want to hear. I could feel the hair rising on my forearms, as though with cold, and rubbed them uneasily—but I took the cigarette and leaned across the table so she could light it for me. I fixed my attention on an old Chinese couple sitting at the next table. They'd barely spoken to one another since they arrived.

"You wonder why Daddy and I got married? I was pregnant,

that's why. We got married because we had to. I was recovering from a broken heart from Eldon, the boy back in Pittsburgh, who I thought I could never live without. Your father was playing at the *Hi Ho Club* in Washington when we met. I was working for the government and we were both living at Shannon's Boarding House downtown. When I found out I was pregnant he had already moved back to New York and I didn't want to tell him, but, of course, I had no choice. It was Ninny who found him in New York and told him. He came back and we got married. Ninny and Uncle Charlie came with us. They were the only ones who knew. When your brother was born I did everything I could think of to make it work, even named him Edward Rutledge Jr., certainly nothing a nice Jewish girl like me would usually do. I bought a Christmas tree, even celebrated Christmas. When the baby died I thought it was my fault. I found him in his crib when he was three months old, just lying there, not moving, dead. Nobody ever really knew why. The doctor told me to get pregnant again, right away, kind of like having a replacement child. That was you."

Of course I already knew the part about my brother's death. That was family folklore. But Mom, who colored in all her life stories with amazing details, had always left that one a little vague. We both knew the point of her confession today was not about the tragic loss that she endured, but her way of telling me, after fifteen years, that she, too had become pregnant before marriage. I never knew why she chose this time to reveal this to me. I couldn't help but think of my own life and wonder if behavior, like an heirloom, could be passed from one generation to another.

Sitting across the table from her, I didn't blink, nor make the slightest movement. For a while we both remained motionless. She stared at me and I stared at the Chinese couple.

"Why are you telling me this now?" I said finally, the words coming out the side of my mouth. If I unclenched my fist I might knock the teacups to the floor.

"There's something else," she said, "Something I never told you. After you, before Goldie, I got pregnant again."

"What? I don't understand."

"What don't you understand, Patti? I got pregnant again after you, not long enough after you. It was an accident. A girlfriend in Pittsburgh arranged for me to visit a doctor. He did—what he did, and he forgot to remove the catheter from inside me. I lost so much blood I almost died."

I recalled the night that Patsy's friend Diane spent the night in my bedroom. I recalled my mother's efficiency in handling the situation, the way I marveled and ascribed it to her general high level of competence at dealing with life. I remembered the night she and Uncle Charlie and I drove around Baltimore, looking for the friend of a friend who would take away the baby growing inside of me, the way Mom studied me before telling Uncle Charlie to turn the car around and drive back home. And finally, like the soft rumble of an approaching storm, I began to remember the darkness and shame and, worst of all, the loneliness I felt being pregnant at such an early age.

Resentment rose within me like bile. Suddenly, I felt thoroughly sick.

"Why didn't you tell me then, Mom? Why didn't you tell me any of this then, when it would have helped?"

"I don't know, Patti," she said, stretching her arms toward me. "I talked to Ninny about it, and we both thought it wouldn't do any good to tell you. Why bring up old stuff? It happened so long ago, and what difference would it have made? It wouldn't have taken away the pregnancy. Nothing would have been different."

"I might have been different, Mom. Don't you get it? Do you have any idea how I felt? I felt I was a bad person."

"Nobody ever said you were a bad person. I never said that."

"You didn't need to say it! It was everywhere I turned. Remember? I lost my "good girl" status. If you're not a good girl, you're a bad girl!" I was vaguely aware of people staring at our table, and realized I must be crying or screaming or both. The drab beige walls of the restaurant turned orange, became wavy. "You should have told me," I repeated "You had no right to keep it from me."

She covered her face with her hands.

"I'm sorry; maybe it was a mistake. Patti, get a hold of yourself. Calm down. It wasn't easy on any of us. I went around with a spastic colon for two years after that. You weren't the only one who suffered. And, yes, I did have a right. It was my life; it happened to me."

"Everything happens to you," I screamed. "You didn't give that baby up. I did! It was my baby, not yours!"

I pushed back from the table, got to my feet and rushed past the waiter, who stared unapologetically from behind the register. The rain felt good on my face. I stood outside the restaurant until I was thoroughly drenched, careful not to look at Mom inside the window.

After that I guess we settled back into our routine. It was easier to keep the line between then and now firmly drawn. The baby and everything about it was once again buried in a filing cabinet in our memories somewhere. We never revisited it again.

CHAPTER 20

I RECALL ONE SATURDAY MORNING, somewhere in the midst of the seventies, while I was still hanging on to my marriage by a thread, sitting on the edge of my bed staring at the phone as if daring it to ring. And when it did, I knew immediately it was my sister calling. It's not like I got to talk to her that much anymore. Her life was as unpredictable as mine was predictable, and I was never sure where she was at any given time. But there was never any doubt in my mind that it was Goldie's phone call that morning that gave me the courage to make my big move.

It had been about six years since *Laugh-In* had catapulted Goldie to stardom, and her face could now be seen on everything from lunch boxes to magazine covers. Six years should have been plenty time to get used to this, but to tell the truth, I never really did. There was something about standing in line at the grocery store and looking up from a cereal box to see my sister's picture on a tabloid or the cover of *Redbook* that inevitably sent a jolt through my nervous system. In the beginning it had been surreal. The first time I saw her on national television was soon after she had left for New York. Mom had called to tell me that Goldie would be dancing on *The Ed Sullivan Show*, and the whole family was coming over to watch her on TV. When we arrived at the house, Mom had borrowed folding chairs from her neighbor and set them in tight rows, right next to each other, like in a theater. Every time the camera would pan past the line of dancers standing behind Ed Sullivan, everyone would start to yell at once. Mostly we just saw glimpses of her, but that's all we needed to gasp and scream. It had been the most unbelievable night. Mom had made fudge and we kept passing it down the line, starting with Uncle Charlie and Ninny and ending with the cousins and neighbors who lived across the street. Daddy had cancelled his music job so he wouldn't miss it. In all the years after, even the night she won the Academy Award, there was never more pride and excitement than we felt watching that first time on television.

It had taken a long time for each member of my family to find the comfort spot in his or her own skin in responding to Goldie's success. Nobody had any idea how the force of her fame would show up in each of our lives. And it kept changing. Sometimes I tried to act nonchalant about it, like it was no big deal. Other times, if I needed a boost, I'd find a way to wind it into a conversation with someone new in my life who might not have known who my sister was, and other times I felt simply intimidated by the life of my little sister. But as completely different as our paths were, there was always one constant. She was then, and continues to be, the person to whom I tell everything. If anything especially good or bad happens, she gets the call. And I've always believed it was mutual.

So the call on that Saturday morning did not surprise me. Goldie knew more than anyone how unhappy and trapped I was feeling in my life.

"Sissy, just do it," she said. "Just get on a plane and try it out. Nobody says you have to stay forever if it doesn't work out. You can always go home, but you deserve the chance. It's not like you'll be alone. I'll be here. You and the kids can stay here with me until you get settled. With your experience you'll be able to find a job in no time."

Seven weeks later our plane landed at LAX, where, surrounded by Michael, David, Ginger the dog, Clarence the cat, and twelve boxes, I knew the second part of my life had begun.

One of the first things I did when I got to Los Angeles was check the job boards at UCLA. This is where I found a job opening for a counselor at a place called *Casa de Hermandad* in Venice, California. Nothing had ever sounded more exotic to me.

It was a September afternoon when I first met Michael Martinez. I was resigned that my life would never include love again. Comfort maybe, but certainly not passion. I had closed the door on that ancient dream the moment I buckled my seat belt and watched Dulles Airport, and my life in Maryland, become a tiny speck in the horizon.

Michael was ten years younger than I and knew of little else except passion. It included every breath he took.

The day was hot and smoggy as only Los Angeles can be, even in Venice Beach. The air was thick and still that day, and the purple arches that lined Windward Boulevard looked even more faded than they were through the orange haze. A young girl wearing Levi cut-offs and a skimpy polka-dot bra darted out in front of me on roller skates, heading toward the beach; I had to slam on the brakes to avoid hitting her. She never looked back. This place felt as if a carnival had bloomed and then vanished the night before, leaving remnants of acrobats and high-wire acts. I expected to see a marching band turn the corner. The moment I had landed in Los Angeles I felt as though I had entered a Technicolor movie where everything was pushed up a notch from the black-and-white world of Washington, D.C. Hair was long, Bob Dylan was still being quoted, and California was a kaleidoscope of psychedelic Day-Glow colors.

My old yellow Volkswagen sputtered as if it was choking to death as I pulled into the abandoned lot on the corner of Lincoln and Palm. I checked the folder of papers sitting on the front seat to make sure I was at the right place: *Casa de Hermandad*, neatly typed on a piece of paper clipped to the folder. It looked a little seedy. Not exactly what I had expected, but wasn't that the point? I was here to escape expectations. I checked myself in the rear-view mirror and ran my fingers over my hair.

The heat had taken its toll on my wispy strawberry hair, so I swept it into a ponytail, and wondered if my lack of ethnicity would be a problem. I was sure I looked exactly like the East Coast social worker I was, and nothing like a Venice Beach community advocate, whatever that was. The make-up I'd so carefully applied earlier had long ago dripped off my face, so I grabbed a tissue from the box on the floor and dabbed at my brows, removing the final remnants of color. I looked a bit like an Albino. Well, my resume should speak for itself, I thought, trying to bolster what little confidence I had left.

In spite of the heat, I began to tremble uncontrollably — from some unnamed fear, or maybe just exhaustion. I had moved two kids, a dog, and a cat across the country. I had no job and exactly $500 in a checking account. Michael and David were confused and angry, and I knew the worst was yet to come, when the reality set in that they had left behind everything that was familiar to them — except me. I sat in the car and concentrated on breathing. Finally, the words I had retrieved from somewhere, probably one of the shrinks I had begun seeing, began to calm and reassure me: *It wasn't my fault. It wasn't anybody's fault. I have a right to a life, even joy. I am steady — I am steady.* The words echoed inside my head like a nursery rhyme. Life is opening up again to me, everything is available. But even through the words I began to tremble again. I sat inside the hot car and forced myself to look at the graffiti on the seedy little building across the street.

Finally, I worked up the nerve to get out of the car and step into the office. Dirt streaked the storefront window of the large room, casting a greenish tint on the empty receptionist's desk. A tattered poster of huge yellow lemons with black print running across the bottom reading—*When Life Gives You Lemons, Make Lemonade*—hung on the wall. My eyes followed a cockroach the size of a tarantula... making its way along a cracked wall. The room was unmistakably empty, the silence broken only by the noisy air conditioner jammed into a corner. "Hello?" Is anyone home? I'm here about the counselor job." I yelled above the noise. "I'm here for my interview."

Noticing a partitioned-off space in the back of the room, I called again, louder this time. There was more silence, and then a man's voice from somewhere behind the partition said, "Oh, Fuck, I forgot. Sorry. C'mon in, you can hang in here." He walked out from behind the wall as he was speaking, and we looked at each other. "I'm Michael, the program director. I'm sorry, time got away from me. The Feds are trying to cut our budget again, and that means we could be on the street by tomorrow. I got lost in numbers, trying to write a new proposal. I'll probably be here all night."

He was a sturdy-looking Mexican kid: dark hair, dark skin, medium build. He was wearing aviator glasses and had a pencil tucked behind his ear. "You must be Miss—ummm. Hawn," he said, glancing down at the resume I had sent a few days earlier—"the recent escapee from the suburbs. I've been looking forward to meeting you." He spoke softly, with a rhythm that sounded California Spanish to my East Coast ears. "I've been holding your resume aside. Welcome."

"Thanks Michael," I said, holding out my hand. "Please call me Patti." I was surprised at how young he looked. I had expected an older, possibly a grittier, street guy or an ex-junkie. They were the types that often took these jobs. I'd been around the system long enough to know how it worked. State and Federal government offices were flooded with proposals for seed money to start up special-population community programs. They were often begun by people who had sprung out of troubled communities and had little to offer except idealism. They had often been through the system themselves and wanted nothing more than to make a difference. It was a time when everyone wanted to change everything.

"I've looked forward to meeting you, too," I responded, a bit stiffly. "It's nice to put a face to a voice. I'm anxious to begin working as soon as possible. If you'd like, I'll furnish you with some referrals from my previous job back East."

He broke into a grin. " Patti, you got the job. This agency is about to go under and if we don't get somebody who knows what the hell they're doing soon, our work here is going to be over. There's not much, actually not even a job, unless we get this proposal done, but we can write in your own job requirement if you help me do it. Wanna give it a try?" He sounded so earnest I had to smile.

Why not, I thought. It wasn't as if I had anything better to do — and besides, I already knew I kind of liked it here — cockroaches and all. And there was something about this kid — not at all what I'd pictured from the brief description I'd found on the UCLA job board last week. Although he was obviously young, I caught a glimpse of something that I hadn't seen in anyone for a long time. His eyes held mine in a gaze so unflinching it made me look away. I could never imagine eyes like that ever caught in a lie.

"Thanks, Michael, for the immediate vote of confidence. I

Good Girls Don't

guess I'm a little surprised. I didn't expect you to be so young," I blurted. "Of course I'm sure you're not as young as you look. I mean everyone in this city looks younger than they are. Jesus, I'm babbling. What do you say we begin again."

Michael just let me ramble, and then smiled the warmest most open smile I'd ever seen. "I'm 27," he declared without apology. "I guess that's young but I sure don't feel it today. My degree is in Public Service. I was one of those inner-city kids that got pushed through programs quickly. Graduated when I was 17 and went on to get my degree a few years after that. Seems like I've been doing this stuff for a long time. I seem to have a gift for getting money from the Feds, and we need all the help we can get."

Michael was interrupted by a sudden noise that sounded like the clanging of cymbals. The incessant whirring of the air conditioner had come to a halt, and the room was immediately seized by silence.

"Shit," he said under his breath. "That's all I needed today."

Within a few seconds he was on his back, plunging a screwdriver into the filthy contraption. "C'mon over here and hold this thing down for me, will you? It's a little grungy under here, but if you put a little pressure on it I think I can make it work, at least for a while. "

I dropped my unread resume on the table and got down on the floor beside him. The heat had already begun to fill the room, and I could feel the perspiration dripping down my face mixed with a film of gray dirt that was tickling my nose. Soon enough the noisy clanging began again and cool air pumped out of the grid.

"So, what do you think?" he asked, pulling me off the floor. "Do you want the job?"

"Of course," I said, "thanks for asking."

He grabbed a tissue from one of the desks and began dabbing

at my face. "You got a little schmutz on you," he said. "Spit on it."

Suddenly the sound of my own laughter took me by surprise, and for just a minute, everything felt O.K. for the first time in a long time.

The kids were spending the night with Goldie, so I decided to stay at the makeshift office and help Michael out. We worked most of the night, huddled over the dog-eared papers of the proposal. I'm not sure where I pulled the numbers from, but finally at around midnight it began to make sense. I knew the language, and Michael knew the clientele. The kids in Venice who were strung out on drugs, doomed to lives of prison or worse, were so engrained in his world that he knew exactly what they needed to get them through the system, and I knew the protocols that the government funding agencies liked. Together we formed an odd but effective team. It was almost 2 a.m. when I realized how exhausted I was. I looked around at the pile of hamburger wrappers and the plastic cups of Coke that had almost been edged off the table, leaned back in my chair, and yawned.

"You're tired, Patti," Michael murmured, his face buried in a folder. "You've been great, but with a little luck I can probably make it work from here. I've been through all this before. Why don't you call it a night?"

I knew I should. What the hell was I doing here, anyway? I wasn't even sure that I cared all that much about this kind of work anymore, at least not like I used to. These kids would probably be back on the street, overdosing, killing themselves or someone else, with or without this program. What did any of it really matter?

"Maybe you're right," I said. "Call me tomorrow and let me know how you stand. If there's anything else I can do…" I let my voice trail off. "Oh, what the hell, I'll stay. It'll be easier to knock this thing out with the two of us."

"Great," he answered. "I knew you were in it for the long

haul. People like you don't give up easily."

"What does that mean, people like me? You have no idea who I am."

"Women like you don't just pick up and move across country, alone, without a really good reason, without something that drives them. You're pretty much alone, aren't you?"

"What makes you say that?" I asked, beginning to feel irritated with him.

"People your age who spend their lives taking care of unfortunates often are," he said.

"I'm sorry to disappoint you," I said testily, "but I'm not alone. If you had read my resume you would have seen that I have two kids and I also happen to be very good at what I do. My loneliness, or lack thereof, quite frankly, is none of your business." How dare this guy take advantage of me with his armchair psychology? Probably something he learned in some Psych 101 class. What kind of insight could this insolent kid possibly have into me? He doesn't have a clue who I am, I thought, or what I've been through.

"Patti, I'm sorry. I over-spoke," Michael said, scowling at his lack of tact. "It's my problem. Always has been. My mouth runs way faster than my head. And it's always getting me into trouble. It's just that I like you, and I really, really need you. Please forgive my big mouth. You can ask me anything, I mean ANYTHING, about my life."

He picked up the resume that I had dropped on the desk and seemed to be reading it for the first time since I'd arrived. He lifted his eyes at one point to look directly at me, almost as if he was really noticing me for the first time.

"Patti Hawn," he laughed, "the same as the movie star Goldie Hawn. You even spell it like she does," he said, his voice going up in a question mark.

"She's my sister and probably the reason I'm here," I answered.

"Wow. I've never met the sister of a celebrity. Must be pretty cool," he said.

I had become accustomed to people's responses to the news that I had a famous sister, but still, there was always that brief moment in meeting someone new when I felt I had to claim myself apart from her. It often seemed that Goldie's celebrity became the most important thing about me, and I always fought against it defining me.

"I guess it's a lot of things," I answered. "But right now I'm pretty tired, and—actually, you're right about calling it a night. I'm exhausted."

Suddenly my body felt drained of any life force that might have made a pretense of an earlier appearance. Everything about this place was new to me. The old ache was back, right where I'd left it before I walked in here. Right now all I wanted was to be buried deep under the covers of my new double bed—luxurious-ly alone. Sometimes familiarity, even when it's pain, feels easier.

"We've known each less than a day and I've already pissed you off," Michael said, grabbing papers from the table and stuff-ing them into a backpack lying on the floor. "C'mon, I'll walk you out to the parking lot. No, better yet, I'll drive you home and we'll pick up the car in the morning. It's the least I can do."

"That won't be necessary, Michael," I muttered ungracious-ly. "I'm perfectly capable of driving myself. People like me, who move across the country alone, are always capable," I added with an edge of sarcasm.

We walked together to the parking lot, the silence hanging in the thick night air, and when we had almost reached my car, he stopped abruptly and took me into his arms with a giant bear hug that almost knocked me over. "Hey, Patti Hawn, sister of Goldie Hawn, lighten up. You got a great big life to start living out here, and tonight you made a friend. I'll call you tomorrow and we'll talk." He didn't wait for an answer but yelled over his shoulder for me to pay attention to my driving—"There are crazy people out there."

By the time I got home I was deeply tired, exhausted in a bone-weary way. I pulled into the driveway of the small house I'd rented in the San Fernando Valley from Goldie, who had bought it for the sole purpose of housing the kids and me. I gazed at the welcoming light through the window. It was all still so foreign. I kept waiting for the owner to come home and tell me to leave. I recalled the advice that someone had given to me before I left Maryland: "Make yourself a nest. Be sure to create a spot that feels safe and warm. You'll need it." The scent of orange blossoms floated in the night air in soft waves. My shoes sunk in the over-watered lawn as I made my way to the red front door, past the pansies and calla lilies that I'd planted last week. The door opened directly into a small living room, where the streetlight slipped through the blind, painting stripes on the brown shag carpeting. A large potted fichus tree dominated the room, almost obscuring the faded floral couch and matching armchair. With the kids at Goldie's house in Malibu for the night, I had the entire house to myself.

I unzipped my skirt and let it fall to the floor, where it stayed in a heap. I unbuttoned my blouse and fell into bed without washing my face or brushing my teeth. The last thing I remember was a vague memory of the smell of lemons and cigarettes that clung to my body where Michael's arm had touched me.

The doorbell rang. Dazed, I jumped out of bed and went quickly to the front door—pulling my robe tightly over my shoulders, not even bothering to put my arms through the sleeves. It didn't occur to me to look at my watch.

"Who is it?" I yelled at the front door, as though I expected it to answer me. "What do you want?" And then, "Go away," before anyone could respond. I still wasn't sure whether this was morning, a dream, or a continuation of the previous night. I heard a man's voice from the other side.

"Patti, it's me, Michael. Michel Martinez. I have coffee and donuts. Open up. I've come to find out why a woman like you would bring two kids, a dog and a cat all the way across the country. I need to know about a woman like you. There was a pause, and he added, "Even if you are Goldie Hawn's sister." By the time I opened the door we were both laughing.

Michael so effortlessly filled spaces with his laugh that it took no time at all to forget that just the previous day, I'd felt lonely. He had the ability to pull me smack into the moment, leaving no time for past or future. We sat in the tiny living room of my house and chatted for hours about our lives. The more we talked, the more exotic we became to one another. He had been raised in a barrio in East Los Angeles, had eight siblings, and was the only one to finish school. He and his college girlfriend had become leaders in the Chicano student movement on campus. His initial dream of completing law school diminished at about the same rate as his bank account, so they decided to take off for a year in an old Chevy and travel through Mexico. His enthusiasm for his native country was so contagious that when he described the size of the cactus and the color of the water, I felt as though I, too, was a part of this country. Michael had a way of tapping into unspoken fantasies that life had never allowed me to even consider.

On the other hand, my East Coast world held a unique fascination for him. As I rambled on about my marriage to Gregg, my numerous jobs in Washington, and the passion that I, too, had discovered when I finally began working for the Crisis Center back in Maryland, he somehow made me feel newly interesting. It didn't take long for me to reveal my secret about the adoption. His only surprise was that I still held it so close. Having a child out of wedlock held absolutely no stigma for him or his generation. He was a little puzzled over why I hadn't kept the baby, but he never expressed a hint of judgment. I found myself telling Michael details of those years that I had never told anyone.

"After I returned home from the hospital and got turned down by the State Department, I felt so worthless," I confessed. "The only thing I could think of to do was to get married. I guess it didn't much matter to who anymore, I just needed to be Mrs. Somebody. I guess it's time to look at another way to show up in this world," I said.

Michael's eyes never left my face. He listened carefully, the way he did to everything, and the more he did, the more I opened up to him. "It's your time now, Patti," he finally said. "The world is about to change and you seem to have landed smack in the midst of it. I think, for whatever reason, your luck and your timing has finally hit it right." He grabbed my hand and pulled me up from the couch. "C'mon, let me take you to a place where they make home-made tortillas. Consider it the beginning of your re-education plan. Let me show you a little of what California has to offer."

Before long, Michael and I became more than just friends. Although we were an unlikely couple, he was just what I needed at that point. We had nothing in common except what Michael taught me. For the first time in my life I felt as though I had no past and couldn't get enough of my present. We worked together feverishly at *Casa de Hermandad*, finding jobs and housing for returning veterans from Viet Nam, nomads in search of the California dream, or self-professed hippies strung out on angel dust. The doors were open to all, and the people who need us found us: in broken-down cars, on roaring motorcycles, and on roller skates. Venice was a Mecca of pilgrims seeking every aspect of free love, and I soon had become one of them, plunging directly into the midst of it.

Meanwhile, my sons, David, now 8 and Michael 14, were spending more and more time at Goldie's home. While I was discovering peace and love, the boys were often dropped off on Friday and picked up in time for school on Monday. David recalls being driven to third grade in a limousine one morning because I didn't get back in time to retrieve him. He asked the driver to please let him off in a place where he could not be seen. This should have been a clue to the confusion my kids were experiencing in their new world. Their weekends were often spent in a Bel-Air mansion while they lived the rest of the week in a small house in Van Nuys.

Although I tried to keep a semblance of normalcy in our home, I often felt out of control. I was a single mother during a time of few role models, and the roles in my life often felt blurred. It had never occurred to me not to be a Mom. Motherhood was the part of me that, like Cheerios or Christmas, was simply non-negotiable. I had spent so much energy trying to replace my lost child that the thought of never having one I could keep was never an option for me. I had jumped into bad marriages and so-called traditional family life in an attempt to stave off a vague, constant emptiness. Although motherhood drove me my entire life, I was clearly making a mess out of it. I had gone head first into a revolution against sexual repression, racism, and everything that challenged freedom of speech, or women's rights. I believed that humanity had been redefined in the 1960s, and I wanted to be a part of this. It felt like, to me, that nothing would ever be the same again. But I think my kids would have preferred a tuna fish casserole.

Good Girls Don't

Every once in a while life throws you a surprising nugget — a gift that can't be arranged or planned and may seem to come straight out of nowhere. I don't believe it has anything to do with star alignment or who deserves what or even timing. It just happens. I've had a few of these in my lifetime — but none so lovely as a balmy Saturday night in October of 1975. Seems like stuff happens to me in October.

The ocean air was pure California as I drove along Pacific Coast Highway with Malibu stretching ahead of me like a rambling path, daring me to follow it, pulling me into possibilities that I had only dreamed could happen. The windows were all open and the air skimmed my face, both warming and cooling me at the same time.

I touched the key to Goldie's beach house, which was tucked inside the pocket of my jeans, pressed against my thigh. She had smiled when she handed it to me.

"Use it wisely, Sissy," she whispered. "No, forget I said that," she added. "Just have fun."

I pushed back the familiar feeling of guilt that was becoming all too much a part of my life lately. I was having fun, I thought. It seemed as though every other day held some kind of a test of responsibility-vs.-fun. The kids, who were again spending the weekend with my sister, would be fine. They'll just be happy to see me happy, I rationalized. But the truth was, I knew they were struggling with everything new and different and a mom who was gone way too much. I was becoming very adept at pushing away guilt. Didn't all the latest books say that guilt was just a futile, empty emotion? I didn't give too much credence to the possibility that it could be an indicator that maybe I should pull back. I loved everything about my job in Venice — sipping margaritas after work in a noisy Mexican restaurant; mostly, being with Michael. It was as though I had miraculously turned back the clock and I was in my twenties, living a life that had always eluded me. So, here I was, on the way to Goldie's ridiculously romantic beach house, perched on a cliff overlooking the ocean, to meet an exciting young man who would become my lover. I had gone from a frazzled suburban housewife—avoiding bill collectors, married to a man who didn't believe in paying taxes—to a heroine in a romance novel. All in less than three months.

I pulled off the highway into the famous Malibu beachfront, past homes that fronted on the ocean. I drove by huge domed mansions that looked like they belonged in Greek mythology, and Spanish ranch style haciendas large enough for horses to graze in the front yards. Although most of the homes were large and impressive, a few small funky cottages stood defiantly in their midst. Goldie had bought her small house a few years before because of its incredible view and proximity to the sea. It was not yet grand or decorated but I had loved this place from the moment I'd seen it, when we first arrived in California. The kids and I had stayed here before settling into our house in the San Fernando Valley. It felt to me as though it had grown directly out of the earth and nestled into the cliff edge. At night, mystical ocean sounds lulled me into a sleep deeper and more peaceful than any I'd ever felt.

Michael and I were meeting here specifically to make love. There was nothing spontaneous about this. We had made the decision while sitting across from each other in a restaurant one day last week after work. We both agreed without hesitation that it was time. He would bring the food, wine, and a joint, and I would supply the place. I had been consumed during the entire week by fantasies of tonight. I had not slept with anyone but Gregg since we had broken up, and the last years had been less than satisfactory. When I left my marriage I assumed sex would re-enter my life, but none of the endless scenarios played out in my head had included anyone like Michael.

Michael's orange Chevy was already parked in the driveway when I arrived He was sitting in the car obviously lost in something I couldn't see. I rarely got to see him in a quiet state. His body, usually poised for action, appeared even more sensual in stillness. We had spent a great deal of time together over the past couple of months and I had become used to his face. But tonight he seemed changed. His eyes were darker, his Latin heritage more pronounced. His elbow was resting outside the rolled-down window, revealing a glint of his earth-colored skin, smooth and dark. The dusty light outlined his profile, and when he finally looked up and saw me, his eyes were so compelling that I couldn't look away.

We hugged each other as though we hadn't just seen each other yesterday, and then found each other's mouths, and kissed with all the passion nurtured throughout the week. We carried the bags of groceries into the house and flipped on a light, but the beauty of the lovely house was lost. We could have been anywhere. We stripped off our clothes and sank deep into each other's bodies, into an abyss of pleasure that for a moment obscured the dull ache that had been part of me for as long as I could remember. Michael set the tempo of our lovemaking, and when he did, he became my teacher. I had no idea that night, but this was a role he would assume for the next five years.

Much later, hunger overtook us, and I sat at the small kitchen table and watched as Michael grilled steaks and tossed a salad. He lit a joint and handed it to me. I inhaled deeply and allowed the sweet taste of marijuana to soften a moment that could possibly be awkward. For a while I felt shy, like a child. Michael said nothing but worked at cooking. As I watched him navigate the unfamiliar kitchen with his usual competence, it occurred to me that lovemaking was like everything else he did. Whether he was planting a cactus or writing a proposal, it was done thoroughly and completely. I had never been around any man who was so accountable, and it fascinated me. He placed two perfect steaks on plates, handed me one and led me into the bedroom where we crawled under the sheet and ate. Moonlight spread over us like a blanket. We didn't talk much but continued eating, making love, drinking and giggling most of the night. When I finally curled into the curve of his arms, we watched the sun come up together, "I wish this night would never end," I said, feeling tears stab my eyes.

He traced his finger down the small of my back. "Me too," he answered. "Who knows, maybe it doesn't have to."

That morning, driving home through the fog-shrouded canyon, I swung off the road into a glen of oak trees and parked. Standing here on this unfamiliar, arid mountainside, I knew I was no longer the woman who had left Maryland just three months earlier. It somehow didn't frighten me that there was no precedent for what lay ahead of me. I stood for a moment breathing in the foreign scents and sounds, and then did something I hadn't tried since I was a child. I imagined this moment inside a picture frame and pushed it deep inside myself where I vowed I could take it out whenever I chose and never forget it.

Almost a year later, I returned to Maryland. Anyone in the neighborhood could tell you what was going on this Fourth of July at #9 Cleveland Avenue. While the rest of the country was celebrating its 200th birthday, my sister, Goldie, was getting married. And she'd come back home to do it.

By this time Michael and I were a couple, if an unlikely one. I was happier than I'd ever been. Coming home felt both normal and strange. Normal because it was home; strange because it didn't feel that way any more.

Mom still hadn't forgiven me for taking the kids and moving across the country. I had to laugh a little, remembering my therapist at the time reminding me that it was not only time to leave my marriage, but also my mother. And how right he had been.

The first thing I noticed when the cab pulled up in front of the house was the wide-open front door. My parents rarely, if ever, locked their door, but even for them to leave it open to the world was unusual. I tripped over a basket of daisies that had been left on the hallway floor and felt as though I'd walked into a florist shop. Flowers were everywhere. Oversized vases crammed with pink roses on each end table in the living room, yellow daisies spilling over the top of the refrigerator, every corner crammed with vases, baskets, pitchers filled with flowers. I later discovered a tiny bud vase with an orchid on top of the toilet, for crying out loud. Mom was on the phone yelling at the Takoma Park police department. "Jeez, Eddie, I told you, I want a patrol car placed at the end of the street. No—not in the middle; at the end. How the hell do you think you're going to handle keeping the peace in the middle? You know I've paid taxes here for thirty years and …yes; of course you'll get an autograph. I'll make sure personally."

A middle-aged woman with a long gray braid hanging down the middle of her back was wandering around the dining room clutching an oversized bowl of crimson tulips, searching for an empty space to deposit them. Mom, still on the phone, waved her index finger toward a corner on the mantle where the woman gratefully and unceremoniously dropped the bowl.

In the background a voice chirped from the television set, describing the grandeur of the tall ships that had been brought into the Chesapeake Bay in honor of this special Fourth of July, but Mom clearly had no intention of being outdone by anything so mundane as ships. I stepped into the dining room, and when Mom saw me, she dropped the phone, probably hanging up on the police officer. She hugged me and told me that young Michael, who had arrived earlier, needed his pants altered. David, who had spent the summer with Gregg, would get there later.

Mom led me through new French doors out to a new redwood deck that perched above the back yard. Moss-draped baskets hung from every tree, and a stone path had been built at the foot of the steps leading down the length of the yard to a small trellis that had been built where my sister and her groom would say their vows. The back yard was bustling with more people than I'd ever seen in there one time, with last-minute tables and candlesticks being unloaded.

"Have you heard the weather report?" Mom's voice was near frantic. "Rain tomorrow. Not just rain, lots and lots of it. I don't know what we're going to do. Your father had the radio on all night tracking the rainstorm. I didn't sleep for five minutes. I knew it was a risk planning this in July. We have weather here. It's not like California." She started to give me a disparaging look but then remembered that's where I lived now, too, and quickly changed the subject.

When we awoke the following morning, the hint of rain covered the back yard, accompanied by a purplish puff of clouds. Although the wedding was set for 4 p.m., Ninny and Uncle Charlie arrived at 10, fully dressed. Uncle Charlie, who had bought his first new suit in 25 years, had been ready by eight. Ninny arrived with several huge black umbrellas which were placed strategically on the dining room table next to one of the vases.

"An outdoor wedding in July? What kind of craziness is that? What were you thinking, Laura?"

Mom shoved a cup of coffee at Ninny, who by then had seated herself in the back room to wait, practically daring the rain to come.

At precisely 3:30 p.m. the rabbi arrived. He said nothing but looked nervously at the sky. Five minutes later the Priest walked in. Since Goldie's fiancé was Catholic, Mom had somehow—we still don't know how—found both clergymen to officiate. They warmly shook hands. But the clouds, even darker now, began to drip fat drops on the guests already seated in the back yard.

Daddy, undaunted, was the first to step out onto the deck. Dressed in his black tuxedo, a white rose in his lapel, he pulled out his violin and began to play *The Wedding March*. His beautiful music, so soulfully played, defied anyone to move, even though the intermittent drops were increasing. And then, at just the moment Daddy finished and lowered his fiddle and Goldie appeared in the doorway, the sun burst out splashing across her face. She was as radiant as any bride has ever been. Her creamy satin gown had been designed to caress her beautiful body, now eight months pregnant, falling softly around her belly like a halo. Daddy took her arm and led her down the aisle.

I followed Daddy and Goldie down the stone path and stood underneath the canopy, waiting for my sister to hand me her cascading bouquet of white roses, so she could kiss the groom. I couldn't help but think back fifteen years to my wedding to Erik. The differences were staggering. The nation may have been celebrating 200 years of freedom that day, but nobody was more aware of how quickly and dramatically things can change than I was that afternoon at my sister's wedding. I couldn't help but think how different my own life might have been if it had not been interrupted by a teen pregnancy, or if I'd married Robert, or kept the baby. It became clear to me that day that so many decisions that altered my life had been made while living on the precipice of radical change.

When I returned to California after Goldie's wedding to resume my new life, it was with a deep conviction that I had made the right decision in moving here. Michael was at the airport to greet us and for the first time, I felt that I was home.

Michael and I spent the next five years sharing our lives. We worked together, creating a program that became a model for community advocacy efforts throughout the city. In our gentle love, I found a peace that had eluded me most of my life. And we both knew when it was time to move on. Michael wanted children of his own, and our love affair was one that had never included the possibility of marriage. My sons continued to need more than Michael could provide for them, and it became clear that our time together was coming to a close. He helped the kids and I move me into a great little apartment in Manhattan Beach, just a few blocks away from the beach. We both knew that it was time for both of us to "get on with our lives." And we did.

It was a couple of years later that I received a shattering phone call from a woman I didn't know, a detached voice on the other end of the line. She informed me that Michael was dead. I felt a searing pain. All I could allow into my brain was that I must get back to the crossword puzzle I'd been doing at the kitchen table. I dragged the phone over and stared at the tiny blocks of inked letters printed on the newspaper. The voice was young, high-pitched…. annoying. Why did it continue to repeat these ridiculous words? Michael couldn't possibly be dead.

"Who are you? Why do you say this to me?" The voice dared intrude on my crossword puzzle. You can't be dead, I thought. You grew bromeliads, painted pictures of purple mountains, made fish tacos and photographed sunsets. I loved you.

"Umm, I worked with him," the voice continued. "He told me about you. I thought you'd want to know. It had to do with the accident. You knew about the accident, didn't you?" Not waiting for a reply, she continued, "Michael was leaving a convenience store one evening and was attacked by a random drug addict. He lost his eye. While he was in the hospital they learned he had diabetes, and within a year he suffered a seizure and died."

Good Girls Don't

I carefully replaced the receiver and stood at the sink, staring out the window at a cobweb on the porch. A fragile breeze disturbed its lacy network but it remained unbroken and continued to stretch and pull. My breath was noisy, out of tune, like a discordant violin that screeched in my brain. "Michael is dead." The words came together to form a sentence. Dead is not an abstraction. It is not a thought or a dream or a metaphor. It is brilliant and garish like the colors in Wal-Mart.

I thought: The memory of you that I kept safely tucked away does not glare and hurt. It was young and beautiful, like you on the glorious day in Venice when my new life began and you returned me to innocence. So many years since we touched, but my flesh still sings when I remember. You cannot be dead. I will not remember you dead. Your smile alone defies death. Your terra cotta skin and chestnut Latin eyes fill with the passion of your music….your art, the sea, the desert. You are the most alive person I've ever known. Although our time together ended years ago, our love remains constant. I will not let you be dead.

CHAPTER 21

AFTER MICHAEL'S DEATH I tried unsuccessfully to fill the void that had taken up permanent residence inside my gut. By 1985 I was franticly filling that emptiness with men who moved in and out of my life as though they were choreographed. The rule remained inflexible: never get too close. For as long as I could remember I had been plagued with a vague lack of connection to the people in my life. My antidote was to keep running in a dozen directions, arriving nowhere, all the while successfully keeping the demons at my back, always mindful to stay one step ahead of the chase. It was exhausting at times, but I'd grown used to this philosophy; there were periods when it actually worked — and almost felt like fun. That is, until things got too quiet. For a time I felt invincible — or so I thought.

One day the fun came to a screeching halt. My doctor had found an unexplained mass on my remaining ovary, and I was whisked into emergency surgery. Fortunately the condition turned out not to be life-threatening, but initially I didn't know this. I had to take a leave of absence from my job and stay at home for a month — a time of imposed, unusual quiet. For the first time in a long time, the normal distractions were out of reach. I was forced

Good Girls Don't

to take a hard look at my life, and the hole in my gut filled up with a profound sadness. Rather than distracting myself once again with my customary hasty change—a move, a marriage—this time I stayed put, awaiting whatever was to come next. Somehow I suspected it was going to be a whopper.

One Tuesday in September, a couple of weeks after my surgery, I awoke to another unformed day stretching ahead of me like a blank page. I couldn't remember the last time, before my surgery, that I'd been at home in the middle of the week. Instead of being exhilarated by the freedom, though, I felt strangely hollow. Nobody was calling me into a meeting about budget cuts or an impending crisis that might alter our program's goals. By this time I was directing a social service program that placed disabled people into jobs and the budget cuts for such services had taken much of the pleasure out of the work. Most of what I did was look for money. There was no man in my life, at least none that I cared about. I did have plenty to be grateful for, particularly my health—but at this moment, as I peeked out the corner of my bedroom window to gaze at the gray ocean, all I could feel was sadness. David had already left for school, so I pulled on a heavy sweater and walked the few short blocks to the ocean to begin my familiar walk. I noted that my energy was returning as I walked the familiar path to the sea. I tried to turn off my mind and just revel in the sheer beauty of the beach, but the more I walked the more jumbled my thoughts became. It became clear to me that I didn't have a clue how to be alone. How in the hell does a normal person have an anxiety attack walking on the beach, I wondered—but that's exactly what was happening to me.

I looked up from the sand and realized I had walked all the way to the next beach town, a couple of blocks from the *Either/Or Bookstore*. I pulled my sweater closer to ward off the bursts of wind that were picking up the sand and sprinkling it into my face like tiny shards of slivered glass. By the time I pushed open the door of the bookstore, I was trembling. The place was empty; the young man sitting behind the wooden counter, lost in a surfing magazine, never looked up. I forced myself to wander to the far end into another room. Within a few minutes I could feel my breathing return to normal. I recalled in perfect detail the day, so many years ago, when I was a pregnant teenager in Pittsburgh, and how I had found solace in libraries and bookstores.

I allowed the musty smells of beach and books to sooth me as I wandered in and out of alcoves that held oak shelves where the hundreds of books were crammed to the ceiling. I let my fingers trail their covers as though I could absorb the words through touch. I felt oddly protected by their physical presence. Nestling into a big overstuffed chair inside one of the nooks, I looked up to see I'd landed in the travel section. By now I was calm enough to read some of the titles that took me around the world. I was surrounded by books of *England's Historical Castles*, or *Guide to Bed and Breakfasts in Spain*. I spotted a book on Nepal pulled it from the shelf. From the moment I began thumbing its pages and saw the photos of Mt. Everest, I became completely absorbed. The eyes of Nepalese children reached out from the pages and seared their way into my being so that everything else disappeared.

I bought the book and sat up all night devouring it. When I was finished I knew I needed to go to Nepal at any cost, even though I didn't know why. With single-minded purpose, I began to make plans. A close friend moved into my apartment and stayed with David, who was in his last year of high school. Normally I would have waited for him to finish school, but the urgency I felt to take this trip was so compelling that I took a leave of absence from work and was on a plane in two weeks. I had never done anything in my life as compulsive, selfish, or irrational.

From the moment I arrived in Kathmandu I was inside an altered space. I was met by soldiers with rifles, escorted into a bus and driven to a terminal, where I waited in long lines to pass through a series of clearances. I stood in the crush outside the terminal to catch my breath while I waited to be driven to my hotel by someone who had been arranged for by the travel agency. I stepped away from the curb to allow a cow to wander past me while fighting to keep my place. The crowd had swelled, people were pushing and I had to use my elbows to stay rooted. I turned my head aside for relief, closed my eyes, and rocked back and forth.

I saw my name, "Miss Pati," bobbing on top of a pole held aloft on the other side of the street, and waved franticly to a young Nepalese boy standing very still, waiting to be found. "Welcome to Kathmandu, Miss Pati," he said in perfect English, obviously rehearsed. He pointed to an old sedan parked down the road and gestured for me to follow. He tossed my duffel bag across his back, and in a few minutes we were maneuvering through the small, crowded streets of the kingdom of Nepal.

If I had wanted to escape 20th-century madness, there was no question, I had discovered how to do it in this almost medieval environment. Nestled in the cradle of the highest mountain on earth, it is not surprising that Nepal is known as the kingdom where deities mingle with mortals. And I, for one, had never felt more intensely the mingling of my own spirit and my mortality. I was still not entirely clear what had brought me here, but for sure I was about to find out.

Trekking in Nepal in 1985 was not exactly the Club Med vacation that most of my friends were taking that year, but it was the right one for me. From the moment that travel book fell off the shelf into my hands, I began to breathe differently. Maybe it was the part about putting one foot in front of the other all day long, and then turning around and doing it all over again the next day, that appealed to me. I'd read that passage in the book over five times, so it must have spoken to something I needed. My life was wound so tightly, always had been, that I guess I thought if the springs ever uncoiled, I'd probably just catapult into thin air and disappear. The coils were definitely unraveling that day in the bookstore, and I figured if I was destined for time travel, Nepal seemed like a gentle place to land.

The driver dropped me off in front of the Malla Hotel, my home for the next week or so. The hotel was situated next door to the Royal Palace, surrounded by a sprawling garden guarded by two large granite tigers stationed on either side of the entrance. I checked my watch and realized it was earlier than I thought, barely noon. I was escorted to a small room where I quickly shed my clothes, jumped into a modern shower, threw on a clean pair of jeans and a denim shirt and flew out the front door, waving to the tigers in less than fifteen minutes.

Clutching my map I headed straight for Thamel, at the north end of the Old City. In less than an hour I'd jumped back ten centuries, into an atmosphere where I felt the ghosts of hundreds of years lingering around every corner. My senses were exploding like firecrackers.

A monkey on a chain danced in front of a girl about seven or eight; a family stooped in front of a windowless hut cooking a meal over an open fire — the smoke's perfume so thick and rich, I stopped for a moment to breath it in. A thin girl about nine years old, wearing a ragged dress, appeared at my side, smiled shyly, and lifted her hands, unashamed, in a silent plea for money. I dug into my pocket and handed her a coin. "Where you want to go?" the child said, jumping immediately by my side. "I'm your friend." Her father shouted something at her and she skipped away, shaking her head, making a clicking sound. I took a right turn, then a left. The crowds swelled — goats, donkeys, roosters

Good Girls Don't

caught in the jam. Two boys wheeled a cart, sometimes right over people's feet. Beggars held out their arms whining: pleeeze, pleeze. Rickshaws cycled past with laughing tourists in the attached carts, and street peddlers displayed assortments of swords, jewelry, and religious images. The ever-present cows lumbered through the narrow streets with the pride of their sacred Hindu status.

I escaped from the kaleidoscope of the streets into a teahouse located in the center of the market square, took a seat and a deep breath. An old man in an embroidered coat and baggy pants, with a long snow-white ponytail and rimless glasses, peered at me.

"Would you like me to clean your ears, madam?" I turned away but he persisted, pulling out of his coat a pointed tool like a small-sharpened screwdriver.

"Thank you, no," I said firmly.

"It's an important tradition here in Kathmandu," he calmly continued, "It helps you to hear the wisdom of the city."

I moved further away from him and pretended to search for someone expected to join me.

"It's safe," he continued. "See, I do it to myself." He probed the inside of his ear with the strange little device, all the while smiling a bit insanely. I left my table and moved away.

"How much would it be worth to hear the wisdom of the city, maybe your future?" He called louder. "You're an American—you see psychiatrists. You drive in big cars and spend money for your big house. Why not give me money to clean your dirty ears?"

I ran from the café back into the crowd and stood in front of a shop window displaying large false teeth. I was sandwiched between a pile of Buddhist offerings of rice, red powder and yellow flower petals, and the entrance to a three-story wooden temple adorned by Buddhist statues of men and women intertwined in erotic postures. I slipped inside the temple. Immediately I was removed from the clamor of waves of people and cacophony of street sounds into jarring silence. I had to wait for my eyes to adjust to the dark. Taking a seat in a folding chair pushed against the damp wall, I stared straight ahead for what felt like a long time. I eased the chair close to the doorway so I could make a fast getaway and listened to the sound of my heart beating. I was afraid it was so loud I would cause attention to myself. A group of three young monks dressed in saffron robes sat on the floor, their heads bowed, obviously heedless of my presence.

Finally the muscles in my neck unwound a bit and I breathed.

What in God's name has brought me here? I thought. I'm scared, lonely, completely exhausted. I leaned my head against the damp stone wall; it smelled dank, like a musty floor. Closing my eyes, letting the silence surround me, I sat there for a long time trying to make sense out of it all. I wondered what my kids were doing. A stab of guilt pierced me as I registered how thoughtless I'd been to begin this strange odyssey at this time. What if the kids needed me? David was only 17; it was his senior year. They'd probably find me stabbed through the ear in a dark street somewhere and nobody would ever know what happened to me.

I awoke with a start and began to take deep breaths. Lord, God, Mother Nature, someone, I pled silently, unaccustomed to praying. Help me to fill up the hole. Show me why I'm here and what I must do. I'm tired of being sad, and tired of not even minding being sad. Tired of being so unconscious. I don't want to be empty anymore. What's wrong with me? I continued breathing deeply, wanting to feel something. began to feel a beat like a soft pulsing in my chest. I breathed again and the pulsing continued traveling down my arms and warming my face. I didn't care if I was imagining this. For today it was enough.

When I emerged from the temple a little dizzy, I realized night had arrived. The glow from cooking fires made friendly shadows along the side streets softening the darkness. There were still the remnants of a pulse in my throat like a tiny frightened mouse, but for the first time since I'd arrived, the frenzy that had accompanied me was quieter. Christ, I didn't come halfway around the world, spend most of my savings and turn the kids' world upside down, to freak out. I made a decision to let the next month or so unfold and just stay out of the way of the usual guilt I plastered over everything. I remembered something I'd read recently about becoming a twig in the river. But I'd be a smart twig, not a foolish one. For example, I wouldn't let anyone insert foreign objects into my ears. I shuddered at the thought. That would be a really dumb twig. This actually brought a smile and already I was feeling better, just bone tired. I easily picked up a rickshaw driver, negotiated a price and allowed myself to be driven back to my hotel where I slept for fourteen hours.

I spent the next few days shopping and sightseeing. I outfitted myself in brightly colored hippie skirts and bangle bracelets. I picked up a yak wool sweater for David and a Nepalese hat with streamers that I knew Michael would love. I discovered temples, stupas, Durbar Square. I took a wrong turn around a corner and found myself marching in a parade. Evenings were spent at Valentino's a café in Thamel where I took my meals and where I easily found myself in the midst of a group of international travelers.

Every time I entered this part of the city I felt a swell of fear and excitement. The stones that paved the roads were ancient under my feet and people were swarming in all directions. One turn could put a person on a street without sunlight, and the next you felt as though you were walking in liquid gold.

One day I took my usual seat at Valentino and decided on a meal of vegetables and rice. I was about to order from a young German kid who smiled at me in recognition when I heard a timid voice behind me.

"Excuse me, may I join you?"

"Yes, of course," I answered before I even got a good look at her.

When I turned around I was looking into the eyes of a girl about 28, with long blonde hair falling in ringlets around a face like an angel's. Her eyes were navy blue and she had skin of pale Italian marble. She was wearing the mandatory travel uniform of jeans and t-shirt with something scribbled on the front in Arabic, and was loaded down with a huge backpack with tent poles jutting out of the top. She could have been a model for a fashion magazine, even though her clothes were dusty and she wore no make up. She was as exquisite a creature as I'd ever seen.

"My name is Ingrid," she offered in a little less than perfect English. I detected Swedish. I'd become pretty good at identifying accents over the past few days.

"I'm Patti. American. Are you alone?"

"Yes, I've just arrived from India where I've been for several months. Don 't go," she said emphatically. "I got caught up in the aftermath of Indira Gandhi's assassination and almost couldn't get out of the country. It's good to be here, feels like I've come home."

Then she laughed and said, "Of course you're American. What else could you be? Even when you guys are traveling you never get dirty."

I wasn't sure if I've just been insulted, but decided to laugh. We spent the next two hours sharing our lives. Ingrid had been on the road for almost two years, preferring Asia because it was cheap and because she simply couldn't get enough of it.

"It gets under your skin," she said. "Asia changes you whether you want it to or not. You don't have to do anything, just breathe. Every time I tell myself I should get back home and resume my nursing job, I can't quite leave. There's always something that pulls me around the next bend, and if I return to Sweden, maybe I'll miss it."

"What about your life?" I asked. "Marriage, children, job, family? Don't you miss any of that? Look at you --- you're beautiful. You could probably have anything you want."

"This is what I want. There will be time for all of it for me. But what in the world brings someone like you here? "

"I'm here because, well, I read a book about Nepal," I stammered, "and when I got to the part about trekking in the Himalayas — well, uh, I don't know. It just really turned me on. I kept reading it over and over. The idea of walking up that mountain began to almost obsess me."

It sounded so crazy that I knew anyone back home would have taken measures to have me committed. When I told mom, who was now living in Los Angeles, that I was leaving for Nepal, she looked at me as though I'd just told her I had planned on selling my children and moving to the moon in search of gold.

All she could sputter was "but you can't do that. You have responsibilities. You just simply can't do that."

Of course that cinched it; the next day I bought my tickets. I certainly couldn't tell this young beautiful girl sitting across from me that at my age, I was here because I was rebelling against my mother. Hadn't it been much more than that? My God, I thought, am I really still that fucked up? Am I still making decisions to shock my mother like when I was a kid?

I looked directly into the blue eyes staring across the table at me, waiting for an answer, and blurted out, "You know what Ingrid, I don't have a clue why I'm here. It just seemed like a good idea at the moment. And I haven't had a good idea in a long, long time."

We both burst into laughter that lasted so long the waiter came over and put fresh glasses of water on the table. And then he laughed too.

When finally we caught our breath, Ingrid said, "Sounds to

me like you're in the perfect spot, exactly where you need to be, and someday you'll probably discover whatever it is you've come here to find. We all do eventually."

We closed down the café, staying late into the night. I ended up spilling my life to this young girl, telling her stuff I hadn't thought of in years. By the end of the evening I had the number of a Sherpa guide named Ang, tucked into the inside pocket of my jeans. Ingrid assured me Ang would safely lead me up into the Himalayas. She added that when I returned, I would probably have more questions than answers — but, then added, as an after-thought, "sometimes the questions are more important than the answers — so either way, you win."

Three days later I was sitting in a helicopter with a handful of other travelers and several Nepalese men — tour guides, per-haps, and the only passengers who did not look nervous. I was on my way to meet Ang at Lukla, a staging point for hikers, at about 10,000 feet above sea level. As we flew past the Himalayas, I was caught off guard by the sweeping sensations that overwhelmed me at my first sight of Mt. Everest — unprepared for the moun-tain's sheer presence. It rested on the top of the earth like an emperor's crown: defiant, benevolent, challenging, its white jagged edges slicing through the clouds with the precision of a scalpel. A hush fell over the passengers. Apparently we all felt the peak's compelling authority. Even the Nepalese men grew silent. Although the ride to Lukla was only about 45 minutes long, by the time we landed I felt as though I'd entered into a completely dif-ferent atmosphere, breathing new air.

Ang found me almost as soon as my feet touched the ground. I heard my name echo through the thin air and looked into the face of the young man who would become my lifeline over the next few weeks.

"Good morning, Missy. I am your guide," he said. "I take care of you. No worry."

My first impression was surprise at how young he was. What had I gotten myself into? I'd just put myself into the hands of a kid who couldn't be more that 17 or 18. Then he smiled, and I noticed the crinkles around the corners of his eyes. He effortlessly pitched my heavy bag onto a yak already burdened with supplies and tents. Although his body seemed slight, like a young boy's, he moved with a grace and confidence that contradicted his youth. He apparently spoke little English, but when I mentioned Ingrid's name his eyes lit up mischievously.

"She's my friend," he assured me. "Golden-hair friend. We will be friends too, like Ingrid." He then became all business. "Do what I say and you stay good." He handed me a smooth polished tree branch to use as a walking stick; it fit my body perfectly.

"Now, follow me."

And I did.

Ang took the lead, followed by a longhaired Asian ox burdened with several weeks worth of supplies, that he pulled with a long leather strap. I found a walking spot somewhere between the animal and Ang. We walked this way along a narrow path for several hours toward our first destination, Namche Bazaar. At first I tried to take everything in at once, afraid that if I didn't stop and look every few minutes I'd miss something.

"How long will it take us to get to the next stop, Ang?" I asked, testing his ability to understand English.

He looked back at me, never stopping his steady pace, and shrugged, "not long, Missy, soon enough."

Although I'd already memorized it, I pulled out the crude map I carried in my daypack and studied it intently, as though it would give me some important answer that I must know.

I was quite sure I detected a smile behind his crinkled eyes.

"Two hours, three, what?" I insisted.

Again he shrugged. "You run, I walk. No hurry."

My first life lesson on the mountain was to shut up and walk. A group of children appeared around a bend who giggled when they saw me. They turned around and walked with us for a while, then turned again to resume their journey. Sounds of bells announced the arrival of an approaching donkey or a yak. I mimicked Ang and flattened myself against the side of the mountain to let them pass.

"Namaste," I repeated, echoing Ang, to two women who passed us, carrying heavy loads, gossiping like housewives. Soon I forgot the map in my pocket. The air was clear and cool, but not too cold, like autumn should be. My feet felt light on the path, as again, I mimicked Ang, planting my front foot firmly during the ascent while resting the one in back. I noticed how my skirt billowed around my body like a sensual caress. Colorful prayer flags blew all along the trail and I quickly learned to pass reverently on the right side of the many ceremonial stone mounds, called stupas, and the Buddhist Mani walls containing tablets with prayers carved on them in Tibetan script. The sunlight seemed pure and peace hung in the atmosphere like a gentle scent. We passed a woman and child traveling down the path, stepping aside to allow them room.

"Namaste," Ang greeted her, and she replied the same. There was no other sign of life other than an occasional goat or cow passing by. Ang stopped and pulled a water bottle from his backpack.

"Drink," he commanded. I drank the water even though I didn't feel thirsty.

After several hours we arrived at the outskirts of Namche Bazaar, the commercial hub of the Khumbu District. The road widened as teahouses and rest shelters appeared along the path. Other trekkers began to pass us and soon we were in a village where Ang gathered my papers and negotiated my passport and trekking permit with soldiers stationed along the path. We continued to a clearing with views of the valley below, where Ang motioned for me to sit while he prepared our campsite. Within a few minutes my sleeping tent was assembled and a small discrete toilet tent dug into the earth about 15 feet away. Ang started a campfire, brewed tea and handed me a steaming mug as he prepared our first meal. We hadn't said much but it didn't seem necessary; a warm bond of trust was beginning to form, through just glances and smiles. I climbed into my cozy tent where I fell almost immediately into a dreamless sleep.

———————————

It was early in the evening of day five, two days before we were to reach the monastery at Thyangboche, the highest point that I'd be climbing. According to my guidebook, the monastery was located on a high ridge at 12,716 feet, and although I was in pretty good physical shape, I didn't want to chance it to go higher. I hadn't seen another trekker or group all day. What surprised me was how little time it took before I forgot everything that had been before this day. I sat in a perch that Ang had found for me and watched the last rays of sunlight flood the clearing as he prepared the evening meal. Tonight we were eating cabbage and potato cake with some kind of sauce, and a wonderful mushroom soup, and of course tea. I laughed when I thought of my strange meal and how seldom I noticed what I ate at home. Here, taste and textures of food amazed me. It was also interesting that my body felt no aches or pains and I seemed to be having no trouble with altitude.

I saw Ang look up from his kitchen chores and turned around to stare at the path that we'd just left. I heard nothing, but he stopped what he'd been doing and walked over to the path and waited. Within a minute or so, I, too, heard the clanging of a bell that by now I recognized as the sound announcing a visitor. A woman, carrying an enormous basket strapped to her head, filled with large clay pots, turned the bend approaching us. None of this is unusual except for the expression of despair on her face. She was dressed in the mountain woman's traditional long skirt and brightly striped apron. Her black braid reached down her back and her face was so heavily lined by weather and work that it was impossible to tell her age. Ang ran up the path and said something to her in a sharper voice than I'd heard him use. They spoke for a few minutes, at first rapidly and then slowly drifting off into silence. The old woman bowed her head; he pulled her to him and began stroking her head with such tenderness I had to look away. When Ang returned to the campsite, he looked down at me and shook his head.

"Sagarmatha take many," he said, sitting beside me. "Her son die, four days ago on climb. Very, very brave man. I pray now."

His eyes fell immediately shut and he took my hand and put it inside of his. For Ang, praying was just another way to breathe. We sat like this for a while; when he opened his eyes mine must have still been closed because when I opened them he was already back at the campfire cooking our meal. I was unaware that his hand had slipped away from mine.

The next day we continued walking higher, the path reaching up into colder terrain with fewer travelers. "Tonight," Ang told me, "we shall camp outside a monastery that is over 500 years old." By the time we reached the tiny village of Thame, on the outskirts of the monastery, I felt tired and my head ached, something I hadn't felt before. We stopped in front of a group of Nepalese villagers gathered around a yak that had just arrived from Tibet, the big news of the day. We ate dinner at the home of a Sherpa family, friends of Ang, sitting on the floor by the hearth.

By seven p.m. darkness had settled in. I returned to my tent, layered myself in long wool underwear, sweaters and two pairs of socks, and began to read *The Snow Leopard* by flashlight. I drifted off; when I awoke again it was almost midnight and my head was pounding like a throbbing base drum. Soon the drumbeat seemed to be emanating not from inside my head but from somewhere outside the tent. I lay paralyzed in my sleeping bag afraid to move. I must be dreaming, I thought. The steady sound grew louder. Waves of nausea overtook me. I sucked in my breath, put my hands to my forehead and squeezed my temples as though to empty out the pain. I groped the bag attached to the side of the tent, fished out aspirin and washed it down with huge gulps of water. Shoving my face out of the tent into the freezing night air, I vomited until there was nothing left but dry heaves. As I wiped my mouth on the sleeve of my sweater I heard something else break through the darkness — the saddest sound I'd ever heard: low, heavy chants that moaned and vibrated against the night.

I opened my eyes to Ang standing in front of a blinding morning light.

"Missy, Missy, you must drink," he said, dripping water onto my lips. "It's the mountain sickness, we go quick. Take big steps. Hurry, hurry, we go down. No time. Bad sick."

I pulled myself to standing, using his arm for support. The mountains spun like a carousel, circling around me so fast I had to close my eyes again. Ang pulled me close with one arm while putting my jacket on with the other. He gently sat me against a tree and tied my walking shoes tightly around my ankles, continuing all the while to drip water into my mouth. Every time I felt the ground under my feet give way, his thin but steely arms kept me erect. My lungs felt stuck to the back of my chest and breathing was hard but he grabbed me around the waist and pushed and pulled me down the mountain. We walked like this for hours, stopping often for me to rest. Ang was both tender and strong, insisting I drink and holding my forehead firmly when I vomited, as Mom had done when I was a child. Realizing the urgency of a quick descent to alleviate my altitude sickness, somehow I managed to continue. Besides our frequent rest breaks, we made only one stop, at a village where Ang hired a porter to go back to our campsite to get our supplies.

For the rest of the day, the only thing I fully registered through my sick haze were Ang's hands, which never left me. Finally, satisfied we had descended to a safe place, he removed his sleeping bag from his backpack and threw it on the field where we stayed for the night. He leaned close and zipped me into the down bag and arranged himself beside me. The last thing I remembered was the warmth of his hand on my forehead.

Day went into night without my knowing; apparently I slept for many hours. Vivid, singular dreams rolled through my psyche one after the other without a break. In each dream I was either holding or searching for a baby or a young child. In one I was lost in a jungle and knew my baby was hidden in the hollow of a tree — but when I finally found the tree, all that was left was a blue blanket. In another I was inside an old beat-up Chevrolet I once owned, driving from schools to apartments to a beach in California, again, calling my babies' names. I knew if I just turned into the next place I'd find them, but when I arrived they had just left. Sometimes it was my son Michael I had lost and other times David, crying out in frustration through the haze of the dream. One time when I heard them calling for me I was inside a dingy apartment with my mother at Christmas, with only a scrawny tree and no presents. I comforted Mom, who was crying, holding a doll with a cracked face. These dreams continued, unvarying and unresolved, for some 15 uninterrupted hours — each one more furtive, and terrifying than the last.

When I finally awoke I was confused, exhausted, drenched in perspiration despite the tent's cool interior. Ang must have moved me inside at some point because he was propped up beside me dozing, although he stirred as soon as I opened my eyes. My body felt as though it weighed a thousand pounds, but my head had stopped hurting and the nausea was gone.

"Where is the baby?" I asked, pulling myself upright, grabbing at the sleeping bag. "Hurry, we need to find him right away; he's lost." It took just a second to realize with embarrassment that I was making no sense.

"You good now," Ang said. "Tea make you better, sickness gone. You sleep away mountain fever and now you rest and eat. Only sleep thoughts. No baby."

"Ang, I heard drums and chants in the night. Was I dreaming? They came so close in my tent. Did you hear too?"

"Yes, Missy, prayers for dead climber at monastery. The monks send boy's spirit off Sagarmatha—to home." He gestured toward the direction of Mount Everest and I remembered that Sagarmatha was the Sherpas' name for the great mountain peak. "It's good thing you hear monks prayers. It cleans spirit."

Exhausted, I laid my head back down and closed my eyes, drifting in and out of sleep for the rest of the night. This time there were no dreams, just deep stillness.

It was as though my tired soul had empted its secrets all over the mountains and now needed time until it was ready to fill up again.

When I awoke, Ang had placed a meal of boiled potatoes and eggs beside me. I was so hungry I couldn't get the food down fast enough. It tasted amazing. I offered no argument when he spooned the food into my mouth, allowing myself to be taken care of like a baby.

I spent another day lying in the warm sun, and by the following day it appeared I was fully acclimatized, surprised at my strength. The memories of my dreams faded, leaving a nagging residue almost like an old movie that I wasn't really sure I'd seen.

The next day it was understood between us that we would resume our upward trek; by mid-morning we were back on the trail as though none of this ever happened. Ang, who loved to sing at the top of his voice while we walked, was in a particularly good mood. Although he wasn't a very good singer, he was loud and loved his own sound. Like spur of the moment praying, it was just another of his surprises that I'd grown used to.

"Today I take you to secret place only I know, and soon you know too," Ang said laughing at his joke, obviously pleased with himself.

By now if Ang had told me we were going to climb to the top of Mt. Everest, I'd have just shrugged and followed him.

"Onward, my leader," I said, "I'll follow you anywhere."

Our laughter echoed through the trees, sounding less like a duet than an entire chorus.

We left behind the views of white mountaintops; in their place emerged a shade of iridescent green I had never seen—as though the sun had just come out enough to spotlight everything it touched with glitter dust. I sat in the midst of a meadow surrounded by fir trees dotted with shoots of orange and yellow wildflowers, all framed in puffs of white clouds. Monzo was not so much a village as a place that feels mythical like Brigadoon or Emerald City. I'd been up in the mountains for some two weeks and my eyes had grown used to seeing beauty wherever they fell, but this was different. Somehow this particular combination of light, color and air, maybe my newfound strength, or maybe simply the pleasure of being alive, made me feel like Alice, just landed in Wonderland.

Good Girls Don't

As soon as we arrived I ran off from Ang and perched myself on a rock. Suddenly tears, and then sobs, overtook me. I spent much of the day like this, unable to control myself even if I had wanted to. The tears had been locked away in a dark, ancient vault for a long time. I cried until I thought there were no tears left, and then cried some more. Ingrid's right, I thought: I'll never be the same again. Nepal had cracked me wide open.

Some time later, I looked at my travel diary and realized the date I began that journey was October 18, 1986—exactly thirty years after that day at Doctors Hospital in Washington, D.C., when my first son was born.

CHAPTER 22
_____

WHEN I RETURNED FROM NEPAL, the first thing I did was quit my job although I had no idea what I was going to do. There was some part of me that knew I was ready to shake up my life again and I needed to find different work to do this. The second was to tell Mom.

"You did what?" Mom said, over her mu shu pork. "What in God's name are you thinking of? What will you do? First you run all over the world risking your life to climb a dumb-assed mountain, and then you come home and tell me you're going to leave your job without another one to go to? You've completely lost your mind! How the hell will you earn a living? You're not getting any younger, you know." Mom had pointed out this fact to me during the course of most of my life with predictable regularity. "Are you having one of those mid-life crises that seem to be so trendy these days?" she continued, "Because I'm here to tell you that you can't afford one."

You had to love her. She was the one constant in my life, never sugar-coating anything. She could always be counted on to tell it like it is, at least the way she saw it.

"I'll make some calls," she added in the next breath, already shuffling in her purse for her address book. "Maybe Uncle

Benjamin can find you something in the shoe business. He's been extremely successful. I always thought you would do well in sales. You have a big mouth."

Not only was Uncle Benjamin, who was one of Mom's enormous core group of "trusted old friends," almost 80, but I was sure he had been retired for over twenty years. I was also sure that if Mom called him he would have walked on water for her.

"Mom, it's OK, don't worry, I'll be fine. I've saved a little money and I need to just figure some stuff out," I said, which infuriated her even more.

"Why can't you figure it out and keep your job?" she said. "If you ask me, you're crazy. But to tell you the truth, I've never understood you."

That was the cue for me to change the subject and move on to safer turf; I began asking questions about the family. This usually soothed her.

I looked across the table at her. Even in the harsh fluorescent light, my mother, well into her seventies, retained a youthful air. Although Goldie had bought her a condo in Los Angeles to be closer to us, she never seemed to be completely comfortable in the fashionable neighborhood where she now lived. She did none of the plastic surgery popular with women who lived on the west side in Los Angeles. Her signature scarlet lipstick still perfectly outlined her full lips, and her brown eyes continued to hold a sensual mystery that belied her age. Daddy had been dead for over ten years, and although they'd been separated for the last five years of his life, she never left his hospital bed during the two months before he died. Like many things about my Mom, her marriage held its mysteries up until the end. To my knowledge there had never been another man in her life. But then what did I know?

Sitting here with her today, I couldn't help but remember another lunch at another Chinese restaurant on a rainy afternoon almost twenty years ago, before I moved to Los Angeles. The day that Mom and I had such a terrible argument and I accused her of withholding information about her life from me.

I hadn't thought about that day for a long time, but somehow today I remembered it in a new way. How hard it must have been for Mom, after the death of her baby, to re-live such a hideous time of her life, through me. Who knows what I would have done under the same circumstances. She did what Ninny said to do and I did what she said to do. It was the natural order of things, just the way it was. Secrets and lies were so imbedded in that era that to do anything different was unimaginable. Mom's ill-timed first pregnancy was kept a secret at all cost, even from me, and I perpetuated the secrets by doing the same. In the light of today, the absurdity of this kind of thinking just made me want to comfort mom. I couldn't imagine what her pain and guilt must have been to discover her baby dead in a crib after all that. I wanted to let her know that we simply didn't know better, And that I understood. It was nobody's fault.

"Let's go, "Mom said, pulling out her credit card to pay for lunch. "I'm getting tired. I want to take a nap."

These naps were new. There was something incongruous about my mother sleeping during the day. The thought made me vaguely uncomfortable, reminded me that she was getting old.

"I'll get the check," I said, trying to pull it from her hand.

"Sure," she snapped. "Now that you're unemployed, you're going to start paying for lunch."

She peered out at me over her glasses, giving me one of her famous dark looks, so familiar that I burst out laughing. I don't know why but I reached across the table and squeezed her hand, a gesture so unfamiliar between us that for a minute we were both a little embarrassed. I had a sudden urge to tell her about the dreams I'd been having about babies since I returned from Nepal, but thought better of it. Why open up old wounds? Mom had done the best she could do, and so had I. I picked up the sweater that had fallen from her shoulders to the floor, and gently wrapped it back around her as we walked to the car.

My kids were both out of the house. Michael, who had come out as gay when he was 19, was involved in a full-time relationship with a life partner. And David was off to college in Boulder, Colorado. For the first time since I was a kid I found myself alone. Although the dreams continued on a regular basis, I chose to interpret them as nothing more profound than the aftermath of altitude sickness. And yet Nepal had cracked me wide open, and there were days I felt naked and could almost watch the chunks of armor falling away.

I don't think anyone was more surprised than my sister when she received a call from me asking to visit her on the set of a movie she was making in Los Angeles. As a social worker, I had chosen such a different path—almost in defiance of my sister's stardom—that my request now must have seemed to come out of the blue.

"I need a job," I said. "Maybe there's something I can learn in the movie business."

"Sure," she said, with good humor. "I thought you'd never ask."

I had spent so much time avoiding my sister's world that I'd only been on a movie set once or twice during the many years I'd lived in Los Angeles. It was only after my return from Nepal that it had occurred to me that there was absolutely nothing wrong with using her influence to help me create a new career - which was exactly what she did. Little by little, I was opening up in a new way — and when I did, I could barely believe the series of events that began dramatically altering my life.

CHAPTER 23

IT WAS A PERFECT SUNDAY MORNING, the kind that makes everyone glad they live in southern California: blue sky, warm sun, and fluffy clouds. A morning filled with the promise of optimism, which is exactly how I felt that day. It had taken Steve and me at least three months, since moving into our new house together, to let it sink in that we were the owners.

The living room was strewn with Sunday papers, and a half-empty champagne bottle leaned precariously against the coffee table; the violins of Vivaldi's *Four Seasons* were sounding loudly through the house.

"Turn it up," Steve yelled from the kitchen as he made our morning coffee. "Remember, it's our house, we can do anything we want."

"Mmmm. You smell like Bolivian perfume," I said, walking into the kitchen and nuzzling my face into his fuzzy blue robe. "I love Sundays, I love you, I love you making coffee, and I love our house. Tell me again how it's our house. Will you marry me?"

Steve smiled back at me with a little glint in his eye. "Well, actually, I was just thinking of asking you the same thing." He dropped instantly to one knee, folding himself into that mythological position that has stopped the hearts of women throughout time.

"C'mon. Stop fooling around," I said, trying to pull him to his feet. "You know I'm just kidding. Who needs marriage? It'll spoil everything. You know our deal. We're TICs, Tenants In Common."

Steve pulled me down on the floor next to him and silenced me with a kiss. When we pulled apart, he continued holding my face, staring at me with an almost comical intensity. "Actually, I'm not kidding. I'm ready; you're ready. Let's just do it."

The amazing thing is that somehow I knew he was right—even though every other time I'd gotten to this point in a relationship, it meant I eventually got hurt.

I looked into Steve's kind eyes, unable to speak, unable to look away. I was almost frightened by the lack of dread I felt when he reached his arms around me and hugged me tight. I'd worn that heavy, wary feeling so long it had become a part of me. But being with Steve was like coming home from a long tiring trip, slipping into a fluffy robe and falling into a cozy bed. Still, I couldn't quite shake the vestige of fear, the testament of all my past failures.

I remained silent, still staring up at him. I couldn't think of anything to say, and that, too, frightened me. In the moment, all I could think about were his amazing blue eyes. They were so striking I could actually see the color from across the room. He usually hid behind a mask of sarcastic one-liners and opinionated retorts, but not that day. His eyes were clear, open, and astonishingly earnest. I ran my hands through the tight small curls of his salt-and-pepper hair, which he kept short to avoid looking "like a refugee from the seventies." He was tall, over six feet, and a little too thin, with the beginning of a small potbelly that he sucked in whenever he thought I was looking. The only fashion he ever cared about was his socks, the more ornate the better. He sold stereos and television sets for a living and told everyone that, for him, going to work was like going to a toy store every day. He was the most honest man I'd ever known.

I remembered the exact instant that I had fallen in love with him. We'd flown down to Mexico shortly after we met for a romantic getaway at a resort in Puerto Vallarta. One night, after we'd consumed an abnormally large amount of tequila, we went back to the room for what promised to be a passionate evening. We were in the throes of some particularly intricate sexual moves, the kind that indicated we were clearly still trying to impress each other with all our tricks, when I became instantly and violently ill. I barely made it to the bathroom before I began heaving and making a series of horribly unattractive noises. Worst of all, I was still sober enough to be embarrassed. But it was immediately clear that Steve was no lightweight. He barged right through the closed bathroom door, pressed his hand tenderly over my forehead and told me to just go for it. It was such a simple gesture, and so reassuringly kind. I knew that this man would be in my life for a long time.

We had pooled everything we had to buy our house, the first that either one of us had ever owned, constantly reassuring each other that we didn't need or want marriage. I was not used to this kind of happiness; it was strange to me and oddly unsettling. Everywhere I looked I found perfection. My kids were fine. Michael was happily living with his partner in a beautiful home. David was finishing college and my new career as a movie publicist was taking off; offers were coming in faster than I could fill them. For the first time in my life I could do no wrong. Still, I couldn't quite quell that nagging feeling that something terrible had to be waiting for me around the next corner.

"I love you," I said thickly, pushing through the sadness that hung inside my chest. "I don't want to lose you, not ever. Please be patient with me. I just get so scared and I don't even know why."

Steve stared at me for a long time, and then, with the kind of aching tenderness usually reserved for a hurt child, he said, "I'm not going anywhere. I'll be right here for you as long as you want me. You know that."

Steve's love and consistent patience so thoroughly defeated my demons that we were married on the beach at sunset the following May. Surrounded by over a hundred friends and family, I walked down along the beach in a long white dress, and Steve and I said our vows to each other, making up the words as we went along. I was glad that my Mom got to see me marry a nice Jewish guy before she died.

That night, I lay awake listening to the sounds of the night. A triangle of dogs had taken up a chilling conversation of barks and howls; they sounded almost human, like a group of children playing some sad and soulful game. Though the summer night was warm, a chill ran through me. When I finally did drift off to sleep, I was haunted by a dream—one I'd had many times before—in which I was lost inside a dark and forbidding jungle. I heard a baby crying. He sounded so frightened and lost that I was certain he was in some kind of immediate danger. I began searching frantically, following the sound of his tiny wails until I came to a hollowed-out tree. I reached inside to take him out, but all I found was an old, worn-out blue baby blanket.

Not the next day, but a few weeks later, the memory of the dream, the weight of it, came upon me unexpectedly. The days had passed for Steve and me in a subdued but giddy happiness. As I arranged a bouquet of wildflowers I'd picked while walking in the canyon around our house, a chain of ideas rushed by me so fast they almost passed me by. I had the feeling of reaching after them to pull them back so I could look at them. I felt as though I was standing in front of two mirrors and watching the images reflect back and forth to one another, each having their own conversation.

What if my son, now almost forty years old, wanted to find me? All these years I'd assumed it was a closed subject. But he could be living anywhere in the world. Maybe he needed to find me and couldn't. All this time I'd thought I would never know, but I saw with embarrassing clarity that I was wrong.

I had to lean against the door to steady myself. My thoughts leapt from possibility to possibility, flooding me with so many ideas it was impossible to follow a single thread to anything resembling a conclusion. I'll never know exactly what it was, on that day, that allowed the memories of my life to engulf me with such force. Perhaps the sense of peace that had finally become part of my daily life held more power than I could ever imagine.

I rushed upstairs to my desk and began writing a letter to my son. When I finished, I dialed information and asked the operator for the number of the Jewish Social Service Agency in Washington, D.C. It was far-fetched to think that this organization was still in operation. After all. it was close to forty years since I'd been in touch with them. I was shocked when the voice on the other end of the phone told me the agency did indeed exist, but was now located in Rockville, Maryland. I scribbled the address on a slip of paper and transferred it immediately to the waiting envelope. Rather than waiting for the usual mail pickup, I drove it myself to the post office. A week or two later I received a letter from the agency informing me that the laws regarding the original sealed documents had changed, and I could petition the courts to pursue the identity of my son. I spent the next few months satisfying the conditions of the court to move forward in my pursuit, and within a few months someone called to tell me that my son had been found.

Everything moved so quickly that it wasn't until more than two years later, while chatting with my newfound son, after a beautiful day of bike riding, that I had the time to wonder what power broke down the wall I had erected between myself and the baby I'd given up. I'm not sure of the mechanics, but I knew that it had to do with finally allowing a man to love me and letting myself love back. Somehow, it opened a crack into the dark hidden place that I'd sealed up so long ago.

Good Girls Don't

CHAPTER 24

"YOUR SON IS A CRACK ADDICT. AND A SCHIZOPHRENIC."

The Maryland accent rang against my ears. I grabbed a pencil and began making tight little circles on the back of a gas-bill envelope on top of a heap of papers on my desk.

"He came into my office yesterday with his adoptive mother," the voice continued. "We thought it was a bit odd for a 40-year-old man to bring his mother with him. It was obvious there were problems. He was pretty disheveled, didn't say much. She did most of the talking. It didn't take us long to figure out he had some psychological problems, mostly side affects of anti-psychotic drugs. His mother is almost 80, but real feisty. She climbed up two flights of stairs like a trooper. Anyway, we read him your letter and he wants to meet you."

I stopped hearing the caller's words after that. I thought she said my son's adoptive father had died when he was 17 and after that he had survived through an endless series of hospitalizations, mental problems and medications. I tried to force myself to continue listening.

Mental problems? Could there be some mistake? Could my son have been switched at birth like that story I saw on *60 Minutes*? Was that possible?

The last time I saw him was 40 years ago: he was 24 hours old and had been put into my arms by a nurse with the kindest face I'd ever seen. I remembered he was tightly wrapped in a blue blanket, and although I know everyone says that babies can't see anything for at least a week or so, I was sure he opened up his eyes and looked directly at me. He knew he was looking at his Mom. There had never been a question in my mind about that.

They had all warned me against seeing him then. And poor Mom; she hadn't known what to do when she realized I was pregnant. "It'll be easier this way," she had said. "Like it never happened. My God, Patti, you're so young. You can't possibly give him any of the things he'll need. You're simply not old enough."

Mom had surrounded herself in those days with a prominent Greek chorus of social workers, doctors and family. The chorus chanted this message in benevolent agreement. Mom was not an easy woman with whom to disagree. The chorus always seemed to swell when they got to the part about the baby being assured a wonderful life. I believed them. So did Mom.

I wished the voice on the other end of the phone would shut up. I had always hated that accent. Took me years of conscious effort to eradicate it from my own speech.

"What's his name?" I said.

"David."

The entire Greek chorus took up residence in my chest and the air left my lungs, stuck somewhere around the top of my throat. I whispered his name, barely audible.

"David," I stammered. "But that's my son's name. I mean, my other son, my David, my real son."

Silence on the other end of the phone.

"I'm sorry," I said "I have to hang up now. I have to let this all in; it's a lot, not at all what I was expecting."

I put the receiver back and tried to remember how to breathe again. Still clutching the pencil, I looked down at the desk and saw I'd written "David" all over the paper. He had a name; he existed. Sometimes, the pregnancy, birth, and adoption no longer seemed real. I was so young at the time, and so much had happened since: a lifetime of stories, marriages, kids, divorces, moves, careers. After so many years edges became blurred and this, too, seemed like just another story in my life. But it wasn't just a story I told. I had a baby and I gave him away. I sat back in my chair and let this sink in.

I glanced at the recent picture on my desk that Steve had taken in New York on my birthday. In it, Michael, my oldest, was laughing so hard I could almost hear him, and David was holding two fingers over the head of his beautiful wife, Joie, like devil's horns. What a night it had been. Birthday toasts, too much champagne, so much laughing.

What had the other David been doing that night? The agency woman had mentioned drugs and schizophrenia. What kind of agony had this son of mine endured? Had he known joy? Had he felt love? Had he made love to a woman or longed for a child? Had he ever wondered about me? Who was this man with whom I was inextricably linked? My blood coursed through his body; he shared my genes. I had given him his life, the one that he endured. God only knows why I wrote that letter a year ago. Hadn't I managed to not think about him for almost 40 years?

Beginning this search, I'd been swept up by a new surge of curiosity, by some romantic notion of a meeting in a restaurant with a man—probably a doctor, or maybe an artist—who might look a little like me. Was it vanity and ego that brought me here? Maybe he had children. My God, I was possibly a grandmother. I wouldn't intrude, I thought—maybe just peek into his life for a moment. I certainly didn't need another son; I had two perfectly good ones.

My breath was beginning to return and the smell of coffee

lured me into the kitchen. I got up from my desk and walked through my living room. The sun had just come up and poured through the window, lighting the sunflowers on my coffee table. Steve's jacket was flung over the sofa where he'd dropped it the night before. Maxie, our terrier, was curled up in a tight ball on the chair, his favorite sleeping spot. Sensing me watching him, he moved his tail very slightly. I mindlessly straightened papers on the table and surveyed the gentle order of my home. Everything was the same and nothing was the same. I poured the hot coffee into a large mug and let the steam curl around me, creating a fog. It felt good on my face, softened the morning a little.

I walked to my front door and pushed it open. Sunlight steamed in. I returned to my office, picked up the phone and dialed the number of the social worker. The Greek Chorus sang softly in the background, "You can't see him, you can't touch him, it never happened." The Maryland accent was back, waiting for an indication of what I wanted to do. I took a deep breath.

"When can I meet him?" I asked.

I had to wait three months before I had the opportunity to sit face to face with my son. There were endless phone calls from the adoption agency to determine whether I had any ulterior motives for meeting David that could possibly be perceived as harmful to him. I was asked to participate in an interview with a local social worker to determine my mental stability. Any information that I received about David was sparse and always left me wanting more. The waiting became excruciating. I wrote him a letter and sent it to the adoption agency in the hope of finding out more about him.

Dear David,

I really like your name. I think it means "beloved." I like it so much I used it myself and named my youngest son David. How's that for a coincidence.

As you know I've spoken to the woman from the adoption agency. Those guys have been pretty awesome in helping us through this "getting to know each other" part. I'm sitting here at my computer writing this letter and I must admit it feels sort of strange to put a name to you – after 40 years. Wow…I'm sure you must feel the same way. I know you just had your 40th birthday – those 0 birthdays can be a bitch.

I hope I've been able to answer some of your questions about me. I know they're kind of vague but it's just a start. I've been trying to think of some of the things I'd like to learn about you – so here goes…

> *What makes you smile?*
> *What's your favorite color?*
> *What music do you listen to?*
> *What is your favorite thing to eat?*
> *What makes you mad?*
> *Is there a place you dream of visiting?*
> *What's your favorite TV show?*
> *Do you like the movies?*
> *Do you believe in God?*
> *Do you have a favorite book or magazine?*
> *What's your favorite season of the year?*

Don't get me started. I could go on and on. It's only fair that I answer the same questions for you.

My dog always makes me smile. He's a small white terrier (short for terror) who hasn't a clue he's small. Nobody ever told him he's not a Pit Bull.

I think I mentioned in my first letter that my favorite color is yellow. As a matter of fact I just painted my bedroom yellow. The other night I turned the lights down really low and made my husband sit in the room and feel what it's like to be inside of yellow. He thought I was nuts.

I love music. My father was a musician. I can't play an instrument, although my parents gave me piano lessons and fiddle lessons but

I didn't like to practice. I will, however, sing, at the slightest encouragement, whether anybody wants to listen or not.

My favorite place to sing is in the car – with the windows up – on the top of my voice – to the radio. Lately I've gotten into salsa music but on Sunday mornings I like Strauss waltzes and Vivaldi. I dance to the Strauss waltzes.

I guess when I'm really hungry I always go for Italian food. Pasta and pizza are way up there. I'm always counting calories so I don't eat everything I'd like to but Hagen Daz coffee ice cream is about as good as it gets.

I have a quick temper and can get mad fast. I yell and scream and then it's over. Someone gave me the finger on the road the other day and although I probably deserved it, it really, really made me mad.

I've never been to India, although I love to travel and have been to lots of outrageous places. Travel is a major passion of mine and I'm always trying to figure out a cheap way to get to some exotic place. I was sort of a hippie at one time in my life, I guess more of a weekend hippie, but took great pride in my "hippiedom." I've never lived in another country but have spent time in some far out places like Nepal and Thailand and even went trekking in the Himalayas. I guess that was the most outrageous thing I've ever done. I did it back in 1987.

I see lots and lots of movies. I cry in movies easily. I'm a sucker for chick-flicks and never miss a Woody Allen movie. Even if they're not very good. I've been a movie buff since I was little and my grandparents took me to musicals and my other grandmother took me to westerns every Saturday afternoon. Sometimes I would see two double features in one day. I love anything from the forties, clothes, and music. I'm a serious romanticist and definitely believe in happy endings. As a matter of fact, I'm committed to them.

I believe in God most of the time, but sometimes I'm sort of skeptical. I always want someone to come down from heaven and say something like "Yes, it's true, I saw Him, He does exist, now everybody relax." The truth is, at least for me, life is just too complicated not to have some master designer. Did you ever look inside of a flower and just be blown away by its perfection?

I have so many favorite books I don't know where to begin. My mother gave me a book called A Tree Grows In Brooklyn, when I was 12 years old and I haven't stopped reading since. I can lose myself in novels. I went through a period of "self-help" books, which made me feel good for a short time. They don't often have real lasting results but there are times when feeling good for short periods of time works just fine. I went through a time reading everything about black people and Civil Rights and the Holocaust and New Age philosophies and always travel books. I loved "Gone With The Wind," when I was kid and was convinced I was Scarlett O'Hara for a little too long. I've gone through periods of my life when I don't read but I'm back on a reading binge now. I never seem to have the time for magazines but I love clothes and make up and hair and all kinds of "girl stuff" and get that from magazines. I also love to write.

What I miss most from leaving Maryland is the change of seasons. It has clearly been the biggest "give-up" for me. If I have to choose I guess autumn is my favorite season. I get a feeling, sort of bittersweet, that goes deep inside when I feel the crisp air and see the colors of fall. I've tried to duplicate touching autumn in many places — but nothing is like Maryland in the fall for me.

David, please don't feel like you have to write the great American novel when you answer me. The answers can be as long or as short as you want them to be and I will be just as thrilled to hear from you, if it's something you would like. This is just a way for us to connect a little which is what I would like to happen. I know that life has thrown you some curves and there are challenges facing you now. I feel confident you're going to work through them and maybe having a pen pal, for now, will give you a smile.

Patti

I was shocked when I went to the mailbox a couple of weeks later and found a letter from David. It was the first time I felt truly connected to my son.

Dear Patti,
Sorry I took so long to write but I find it hard talking about myself. My life has been pretty good so far. I grew up in a suburb of Washington,

D.C. My father owned a car wash. He worked hard and I got a pretty strong work ethic. I got Bar Mitzvahed, we are Conservative Jews. I got sent away to boarding school where we meditated and studied Zen Buddhism. It didn't prepare me too well for college but I went anyway and studied Philosophy. The German Idealists were my specialty. College was the best years of my life because I was self-supporting and thinking real good. When I graduated college I hitchhiked around the United States. I jumped freight trains and played the penny whistle, worked off jobs such as bailing hay and dishwashing. During this time I got involved in Orthodox Judaism. My interest in Judaism touched my interest in getting in touch with you. Around five years ago I made a half-hearted attempt to contact you. They gave me a small description and I was satisfied, but now my interest is overwhelming even though I have drifted away from Judaism.

Well, onto your questions.

Groups of people make me smile. I'm used to being alone, but groups make me smile.

My favorite color is Blue. I like sleeping under the clear sky of Texas.

I play penny whistle and like rock and roll. When I was in France I got to play with a band. Vivaldi has always been a favorite of mine. I also like Neil Young.

I like to eat hamburgers and French fries. When I traveled I didn't eat much so anything tastes good to me.

I don't have a temper. I keep it inside most of the time.

It's exciting to hear that you've traveled to the Himalayas. I dream of India, but I am tired of traveling.

I believe in G-d. It came while studying Talmud with the Orthodox people.

I like philosophy books. The more abstract the better.

Autumn is my favorite season. I went to boarding school in NY, along the Hudson River and autumn was the most beautiful.

Sorry I took so long to write, and, yes, it does bring a smile to write to you.

David

CHAPTER 25

My breasts are full. They're tender and swollen and their milk falls in creamy drops onto my belly. Why do you not drink this? It's for you. The mild drops rain from my young breasts, the milk you never drank. They told me it would dry up and disappear but they were wrong. How different your life might have been if you'd tasted the sweet sustenance you were meant to drink. Forgive me.

I WAITED INSIDE THE LOBBY OF an unremarkable office building that replaced the old Jewish Social Service Agency I last visited some forty years ago. Waiting was a thing I'd had lots of experience doing. Waiting for the courts to unseal the adoption papers. Waiting for the results of a mandatory psychological evaluation to make sure I wasn't too crazy. Waiting for the social worker to make sure my son was finally ready to meet me.

All this waiting gave me time to breathe and produced something that felt almost like relief. I felt vaguely surprised by this unexpected patch of mental serenity. It was the last thing I expected to feel, but I gladly accepted it as I sat on the drab brown sofa waiting to meet my son after 40 years.

I concentrated on keeping my hands still, and then I felt a

breeze move through the room from the open window. I walked to it and stared out at the dark fringe of trees that reminded me I was back home in Maryland. It was unseasonably warm for February and the trees were still bald, but they were unmistakably the trees of my youth. I knew that in a month or so pink blossoms would appear on the brittle dogwood and clouds of cherry blossoms would spill out over neighborhoods. I could almost smell them coming.

Voices filtered through closed office doors, rising and falling. I wondered if they were sealing the fates of mothers and their babies inside these offices, like they did mine and David's. Footsteps land on the tiled floor behind me: steady, unhurried steps that knew clearly where they were going. I stood up straighter, taller. The eye of the storm had passed; it was time to get back into the game. My heart was now beating so loudly I could hear it inside my ears.

"Patti, is it you?" It was the now familiar voice of Beth Lundgren, the social worker to whom I'd spoken so often on the phone during the past three months.

"I'm glad to finally meet you in person," I said.

I floated above the scene and looked down to see myself, a young girl, dressed up and doing a poor imitation of a middle-aged woman. Why was my voice all whispery? Fortunately, Beth didn't seem to notice, because she put out her hand and smiled warmly.

"I know this is a big day for you, and we're here to make it as comfortable as possible."

That's when I heard the accent. The one that took me back to 40 years ago, to the voice of Madeleine Greenberg—a memory I'd buried because I hated it with the unreasonable vengeance that only a frightened teen-aged girl could feel. I cleared my throat.

"Is David here yet?"

Good Girls Don't

"He's coming with his counselor from Fellowship House. We thought it would be best if he had support here. We also invited the caseworker from the adoption agency that has been involved in doing the research into David's past."

We climbed the stairs into a small office where six folding chairs had been arranged. I chose the seat furthest away from the others, instinctively claiming space, holding my manila envelope like a shield across my chest. Beth pulled her chair up and placed her hand on mine, dragging her palm over the tops of my fingers. I quickly pulled my hand away, uncomfortable with the intrusion.

The door opened, and before I could react two more people filed into the small room. I was introduced to a middle-aged balding man — a caseworker — and an attractive young woman with billowing dark hair whose identity I never learned.

Then David was there, standing in the doorway with someone behind him. I felt tears gather in the back of my throat. I rose to my feet and everyone in the room disappeared from my view. He was slender and dark. He wore glasses, but they didn't for a moment obscure his brilliant blue eyes. He was dressed in khakis and a white shirt that was only partially tucked in. He took a step or two and I saw that he shuffled, moved as though his joints were stiff.

"I've waited so long to meet you," I said. "May I hug you?"

David said nothing, but smiled. And when he did he was so radiant and his smile so dazzling that I felt blinded by its light. He slid into my arms and the light stabbed my chest, crumbling walls inside of me as if they were made of paper. After forty years of waiting, I felt whole again.

I immediately felt the need to protect him. He appeared vulnerable, like a wounded animal inside this tiny room. I instinctively knew he wasn't used to being the center of attention, and today it was as though we were both actors trapped inside a theater-in-the-round: surrounded, once again, by the Greek Chorus of long ago. My first impulse was to mask any perceived discomfort with the sound of my voice.

"David, " I said, "it's wonderful to meet you. Let me look at you. I think we look alike. I've brought photos of everyone in my family for you to see."

I closed my eyes. "Shut up," I said to myself. "Stop jabbering." What I really wanted to tell David was how sorry I was. Sorry I gave him away. Sorry he was sick. I wanted to explain to him that it wasn't my fault. Nobody in my family had schizophrenia. Maybe I could have saved him from it, though, if only I had kept him — been older, smarter, better. But of course, I said none of these things. Instead, I reached into my purse and pulled out a paperback book of the life of Neil Young and continued to jabber.

"In your letter you mentioned that you liked Neil Young so I brought you this book. Thought you'd get a kick out of it."

David took the book graciously without ever taking his eyes off my face. He was so calm and composed. Why couldn't I stop talking?

"You know," I continued, "I'm going to be here for a few days so maybe we can see each other, have dinner, or lunch or just hang out -- or something. Whatever you'd like. I live at the beach in California but I still have family here, so I come back pretty frequently and — "

"I think I look like you," he interrupted, scrutinizing my face, touching it easily with no trace of self-consciousness. He traced my cheek with the back of his hand in a gesture so gentle, it made my eyes tear up and finally quieted me. We spent the next minute or so openly staring into each other's faces, saying nothing. It was as though an unspoken agreement had taken place between us to drop unnecessary chatter and simply examine one another.

We stayed like this for a while longer. I showed him more pictures of Michael and David and told him about my house in

Manhattan Beach. I was in the middle of telling him about my job as a movie publicist when suddenly he interrupted me mid-sentence, shaking his head in disbelief.

"You're my mother." He murmured. "You're really my mother."

"Yes, David," I said, my voice dropping to a whisper. "This is true. I really am your mother."

David and I made a date for the following day to meet at Fellowship House in Baltimore, the group home for emotionally disturbed people where he lived. Traffic was bumper to bumper all the way back into Silver Spring, but I didn't mind. I maneuvered my car onto the Washington Beltway, actually relieved to have the time. I needed to try and fit the pieces of David's life together so they made some kind of sense to me. It felt like an impossibly difficult jigsaw puzzle. I had no idea where to begin. I went over the facts in my mind—stuff I'd learned from Beth—and tried to arrange them in some sense of order.

I began by imagining David at twelve, which wasn't hard to do after meeting him today. I could see how he might have looked as a child: he might have worn thick glasses; probably was slight, small for his age. Beth said he began using LSD at this extraordinarily early age. Why would a kid from a seemingly traditional Jewish family in the suburbs in the early seventies turn to such drastic experimentation? I did some quick arithmetic in my head and realized that was exactly the time when I began working as a drug counselor at the crisis center in Silver Spring. I recalled the steady stream of frightened parents desperate for answers and their reluctant, sullen kids in tow. A shudder ran through my body. My God, David could have easily been one of those kids. David's parents addressed the problem by sending him to a boarding school in Poughkeepsie, New York, from which he came home only sporadically. I don't think he lived at home much after that.

I recalled the letter I wrote his mother after I'd received word that David had been found. Beth had told me that the mother was older than I by almost twenty years, and that her husband had died when David was seventeen. I took such great care writing that letter, which was essentially a thank-you note—acknowledging the daunting job she had been given, assuring her that I would never intrude on their family, or for that matter, on David. I was disappointed she'd never responded.

I couldn't help but think of the synchronicity between David's 40th birthday and the call he received from the agency letting him know that I was looking for him. Both events occurred at a moment when his life had plummeted into crisis. It was the very day he went to court to be sentenced for shoplifting a box of laundry detergent, and had then been placed on probation to Fellowship House.

Driving back to Takoma Park after our first meeting I stared out at the highway, felt my eyes filling with tears as I pulled off onto a rural service road, blinking quickly to improve my vision. I desperately wanted to reach back in time and snatch this little boy away from boarding school and drugs and what felt to me like certain loneliness. As my chest tightened with an intense sadness, I tried to give myself some comfort.

I searched my mind for the next event of David's life. If I could just put these facts in order, maybe I could control the rush of painful images of David—tripping on drugs, lonely and far away from home—that had begun to flood over me. He graduated from Clark University in Worcester, Massachusetts, with a degree in philosophy. After that the information became sketchy. Apparently, he began what sounded like a nomadic existence, traveling all over the country. He'd even gone to faraway places like France and a kibbutz in Israel.

I'm not sure when he had his first psychotic break, or if that's what it actually was. Beth told me that he'd been hospitalized at least twice for long periods. Somebody along the way must have declared him a schizophrenic and put him on medication. During my years in social work, I had often seen this diagnosis used when none other could be found, and I wondered how accurate it was. Could he have just been depressed or scared?

The last ten years of his life were relatively stable — until this latest relapse. He spent it working not far from where I was raised and living in an apartment bought for him by his mother.

I looked up and realized the service road had dropped me off in a thicket of bare, shivering oak trees. It was twilight, the sun had begun to set and the cool air had sucked the early promise of spring from the day, but I decided to get out of the car anyway. A few feet away, a creek meandered through the woods and I was reminded of Sligo Creek, the one that ran close to my house when I was a child — my place of refuge when I was sad or angry. Looking at the creek, feeling the air and smells of my childhood around me, I was suddenly fifteen again, in the back of my house waiting for Mom to find me, to tell me what to do.

The following morning, I arrived in Baltimore half an hour earlier than planned and, as I have so many times in my journey with David, found myself inside a waiting room. Fellowship House was a freshly painted brownstone in a tree-shaded residential area, away from the bustle of the Baltimore harbor.

It was Saturday morning, and from my view inside the waiting room, the place looked a little like a busy college dormitory. Every once in a while someone walked by to peer in at me. One young girl, who at first glance looked like she might have been off to a high-school football game, wandered into the room and stared at me, making no effort to mask her intense curiosity.

"Who're you?"

When I answered that I was waiting for David, she didn't respond but continued to scrutinize me.

"How old are you?" Before I could answer she plopped down next to me and began stroking my leather jacket. "It's so soft," she crooned, "Feels smooth, nice. What's your name?"

"Patti. What's yours?"

"Oh, I know who you are," she said again ignoring my question. "You're the lady who found David. You gave him away a long time ago and now you've come to get him. He told us last night at the group meeting. You're nice. David says you're nice."

A young man who I recognized from the earlier meeting with David appeared and told my young companion that her group was about to go grocery shopping, that they were waiting for her. I waved but she was gone before I could say goodbye.

The counselor, whose name I remembered was Bob, ushered me inside a warm, comfortable office where I settled into a leather armchair, eager to learn anything that I could about David before he arrived. I noticed that the paint around the window was peeling and the desk was propped up on one side by a couple of books where the leg had broken off. I later learned that the funding necessary to keep the place going was in jeopardy.

"Meeting you has been terrific for David," Bob began. "When we came back last night he told everyone at the group meeting about it. It was the first time he actually opened up."

"How much do you know of David's medical history?" I asked.

"Not much. Seems he was pretty stable for a long time before this last crisis. His mom was happy when I got him sent here instead of jail, that's for sure. She's sure energetic for an old lady."

He chortled thoughtfully. "Almost eighty."

Bob told me that when David first came to the Fellowship House, he had a job in a factory, putting labels on cans for minimum wage.

"Used to get up before dawn every morning to catch all the right buses to get there. Took two hours each way. But when his boss found out about David's history, he let him go. I'll tell you one thing, though. The guy's got one helluva work ethic."

Bob frowned a little. "I think David may have slipped through the cracks, though. I've been hired by his mother to help get him services, but he's older than most of the people just finding their way into the mainstream of the rehabilitation maze." He shrugged. "We're doing our best."

There was something about his tone — offhand and slightly flippant — that irritated me. I might have to tell him that I, too, had worked in the system, so that he'd drop the cynical-but-hardy social-worker posture.

We both looked at our watches and realized that David was close to 45 minutes late. Bob said he had seen him earlier in the morning on his way out for coffee, and I sensed his dawning discomfort.

"Can't imagine what's taking him so long," he offered weakly. "He was really excited about today."

"Do you think anything's wrong?"

"No, no, I'm sure he'll be here. David sometimes has problems with timelines," he added, checking his watch again. "But I admit I am a little surprised."

I felt my heart sink. Maybe David didn't like me. I probably came on too strong, overwhelmed him. The possibility of actual rejection reared its head, something I'd either not considered or kept back in the shadows of consciousness. As I teetered on this precipice of self-criticism and panic, my son arrived looking particularly disheveled.

Bob's schedule had been rescued, but he was not about to forgive David for the scare.

"David, we've been waiting for you. Patti's been here for an hour," he said impatiently. "You must always remember to let us know where you go." It was as though he was speaking to an errant child.

"I'm sorry I'm late," David said, hanging his 40-year-old head. "Must've lost track of time. Sorry."

I sucked in my breath and resisted telling Bob to lighten up. I'd only known David for 24 hours and I was already poised to fight his playground battles for him.

Today when I saw him I fought a strange, almost primal urge to touch him. I certainly didn't want to embarrass either one of us, but it was so intense that I could barely contain myself from walking across the room and latching onto his arm.

"Forget it," I said to David. "I got a chance to talk to Bob and got filled in on all your secrets. C'mon, let's get out of here. Show me Baltimore."

I grazed David's shoulder as I walked by him and gratefully noticed that he made no move to resist my touch. He did, however, look at me as though he was not sure how to take me. Then he laughed a big jolly laugh that was surprising coming from his slight frame. The sound and resonance of it awakened a memory from a long time ago: I was dropped directly into the moment when I first met his father on that October morning so many years ago when the school bus dropped me off for my first day of high school. I let David take the lead, winding us through back streets and alleys toward the harbor. I took a chance and grabbed his arm to let him lead me across the street, and was immediately struck by the comfort I felt in his physical presence. At the same time, I noticed that his arm felt thin and stiff through his worn jacket, which was stained with smudges of ground-in dirt, and that his

Good Girls Don't

pants were too long; they fell way below his heels and dragged on the pavement.

It was cool, if still warm for February, and the chilled air felt clean on my face. I resisted the urge to fill up space with words and made myself content to just walk beside him. As hard as it was to believe, there was something almost regal about David's presence. He was oblivious to the odd looks that we got from people we passed along the way, and soon I didn't see them either.

I glanced at David and tried to examine him without being too obvious. On the surface we seemed so different. His olive complexion and thick dark hair were the complete opposite of my fair skin and light hair. I thought he looked younger than his age, despite the fact that he wore thick glasses and his teeth were badly stained. And I noticed he had an unconscious habit of moving his jaw from one side to the other in a rather exaggerated yawn and that he swallowed often, almost as though he was gulping for air. Still, there was something that definitely tied me physically to this man. The shape of his face; his startling blue eyes. For a moment I saw him as he might have been without the side effects of Prolyxin, the anti-psychotic drug he'd taken for so many years.

I realized I was holding his hand too tightly, but when I tried to release my grip he continued to hold on. Almost as though on cue, we both studied each other's fingers, placing our hands together as though to measure them against each other. I'd always hated my hands. My fingers were short and flat with wide nails, like those of a peasant woman. And my little finger barely reached past the first knuckle of my ring finger. My mother used to tell me I got my hands from my grandfather, as if that fact alone was reason enough to love them. David's hands were exactly like mine. We laughed at the uncanny similarity of our funny, stubby fingers, holding our hands tightly against each other.

"A gift from my grandfather," I said, as we continued to

regard each other's hands. "Speaking of grandfathers, your grandfather, my dad, was a very talented violinist. Do you play an instrument?"

"I used to play the penny whistle."

I wasn't at all sure what a penny whistle was but made an instant decision to let that one go until later. I had to be careful not to bombard him with questions. How do you start to fill in so many years? Maybe you don't. Perhaps you don't force the issue; you just let it happen, I thought, knowing I was probably incapable of exercising that kind of restraint.

"I never learned to play anything, but I used to take dancing lessons."

He nodded.

"OK," I said, giving up. "What's a penny whistle?"

"It's a tin whistle, like a recorder," he said, offering no other information. I nodded, as though I understood. I was beginning to pick up on his rhythm. I said many sentences and he said a few words. I convinced myself that, somehow, it was working.

We passed a homeless man on the street and David broke away from me, reached into his pocket and pressed a coin into the man's hand. These two men stood together in the cold street, and they were briefly interchangeable. There was almost an unspoken understanding between them that transcended words — maybe something like, "today I give the coin, tomorrow I get the coin." We continued wordlessly, walking briskly in perfect rhythm. It was David who finally broke the silence.

"Are you here on business?" he asked.

Not what I was expecting. Was he testing me?

"David, don't you get it? I'm here to see you. I came from Los Angeles to meet you." I spelled it out slowly. "I've been looking for you for a long time. Nothing, absolutely nothing to do with business."

He smiled slowly, and then nodded.

We ducked into one of the busy tourist restaurants that lined the harbor. I ordered a crab cake sandwich and he did exactly the same.

"I have so many questions," I began. "Shall I ask them, or wait? Do I pry too much?"

"I don't mind. Ask anything. It's a good thing one of us talks."

"The medication. Has anyone changed it lately?"

"No. It took me a long time to agree to take it. I hated it, but now I don't care so much. It's been so long. I guess I'm used to it."

"Tell me about your family."

"My father died suddenly of a heart attack while we were on a family vacation in Florida. I was seventeen. It was horrible. I think my brother blamed me because I was always the one in trouble. He, my father, owned car washes. Lots of them. Always worked long hours. Guess I really never knew him all that much, but I learned my work ethic from him."

"Why did you go away to boarding school, so young? Were you really only twelve? Wasn't it lonely?"

"I guess my parents felt it was best for me. Besides, I liked it. There was a teacher, we became friends. It was OK."

I knew I was taking huge liberties, treading dangerously, by asking him such direct and confrontational questions, but I couldn't stop myself.

"What about the drugs? The illegal ones, the crack? I hope you don't mind me asking you but, Jesus, David, you have to know. I've been looking for you for a long time and I sure don't want to lose you now to something like that."

"It was really, really stupid. I got in with a bunch of people that used to hang around the deli in Langley Park, where I worked for ten years. I've always been a loner, but for a while I didn't feel alone and I liked the feeling. I'm not even sure how it happened, but it did. It was awful, like a downward spiral that I couldn't get out of. I lost my job, my apartment, everything. It's over now."

I shook my head. I had been a drug counselor for quite a few years before I moved to Los Angeles. I worked with kids strung out on every drug imaginable. I had heard all the stories, reasons, promises, and I knew the realities better than most. But when David told me this I believed him. Even though I told myself not to, I did.

"Your Mom, what's she like?"

"She takes care of me," he stated simply. "And, she plays mah jong. I call her every Sunday. Always have. What do your kids do?"

Something told me this question was important to David; he was not just making conversation.

"Michael works for a doctor and David is a chiropractor."

I tried to match his short, straightforward style. I was not at all sure why, but I didn't want to talk about my kids. I'd rather keep this on him. I was afraid he'd ask me questions I wouldn't know how to answer. Didn't want to answer.

"How old are they?" he persisted.

"Michael was not much younger than you. David, the other David, is 30."

"Did you ever consider an abortion when you were pregnant with Michael?"

His question left me nearly speechless. I reminded myself to swallow.

"No."

Where did that question come from? I would not have been surprised if he'd asked me if I'd considered an abortion when I was pregnant with him, but why Michael? Was this David's way of saying to me, "why him and not me?" Did he mean that giving him up was akin to an abortion? I felt sickened by the question, and more so by the rush of painful memories that followed.

David and I spent the rest of the day walking aimlessly for hours, sometimes silently, other times lost in conversation. I paid for lunch and was surprised by how formal he sounded when he thanked me. It seemed he took nothing for granted. At one point during the day he interrupted something I was telling him to share a dream that he'd had the previous night. It was the first time he showed even a hint of animation. We were sitting at a café having coffee and his voice became loud enough to cause a young woman sitting at the café with her children to look up at us, an alarmed expression on her face.

"I dreamed I killed a security guard last night," he said.

"What do you think it meant?" I asked.

"I guess something to do with meeting you. I don't know."

I showed him the pictures I've brought, which he carefully studied as though to memorize them. I'd chosen each photo with care—pictures of my mom and dad, me and my sons. I'd purposely left out any images that included Goldie, having made the decision to wait on that subject. I pulled out a prom picture of Robert in his white dinner jacket and me in my pale-green tulle ballerina gown, taken so long ago. David examined the photo closely but said nothing.

"I think he's a nice guy," I said. "But I'm not real sure. I know that he got his Ph.D. and eventually retired from the Air Force. I heard he became the president of a small college down south. Do you want to meet him?"

"Very much," he answered. "I was a philosophy major in college, too."

He hesitated and seemed to be on the verge of saying more, but then lapsed into silence.

"I'll find him," I blurted out. "I found you, didn't I?"

"Why?"

"Why what?"

"Never mind." He pointed to the picture of Robert: "Will you tell him about my problems?"

"I don't know," I said, taking my time. "Before we met, all I would have been able to tell him was what was on paper, and you can't really know someone by that. Now that I've seen you smile and heard you speak, I'll have something to really tell him about."

David grinned and his large eyes become even bigger; they just knocked me out. They were an amazing shade of blue, like chunks of sapphire, and they crinkled up at the corner when he laughed.

As we walked back to Fellowship House, I couldn't stop thinking about the question he stopped himself from asking: "Why?" I wondered if he wanted to know why I tried to find him, or why I gave him up in the first place, or—and my stomach turned—why I waited so long track him down. As I chewed on these questions, I had a vague realization of something put off, something needing to be done, and the taste in my mouth was of shame and resolve.

It was dusk when we got back to Fellowship House. David asked Bob to take a picture of us sitting on the stoop together, and I felt the strength of both of his arms wrapped around my shoulders. I felt good knowing that he, too, shared my desire for touch. We walked arm in arm to the parking lot, and when I turned to reassure him that I'd return, I saw his eyes brimming with tears. Before I could speak, he cupped my face in his hands and gently kissed me.

Good Girls Don't

CHAPTER 26

AFTER I RETURNED HOME FROM BALTIMORE I went about the business of finding Robert Marsden. It wasn't that hard. People often have said to me they have to die to get out of my life.

I'd been sitting at my desk for twenty minutes, staring at Robert's number, trying to remember the last time I'd seen him. We had run into each other at a ten-year high school reunion: his, not mine. Patsy had insisted that I go, reminding me that her class had been more like mine than my own and told me, as an afterthought, that she'd heard Robert would be there. She told me at the time that he was a pilot in the Air Force—had just returned from Viet Nam and was coming home to deliver a memorial eulogy for one of his classmates who had died in a plane crash over Hanoi.

I was heavily involved in the anti-war movement then; I had actually been arrested during one of the protests. Thus, when Robert entered the Manor Country Club dressed in full Air Force regalia, I was less than impressed. What surprised me most about this memory was how coldly I had extricated him from having anything to do with my pregnancy. In fact, I was barely able to remember anything about that evening except disdain for his politics and the strange dance we shared: me braless, wearing a micro-mini-skirt, and he in full dress whites with a huge saber dangling from his belt.

I dialed the number that my old friend Patsy had found for me and asked a woman with a distinctively Southern accent to connect me to Dr. Marsden. Patsy was one of the first people I had called after I found David. It took exactly one day for her to get back to me with Robert's phone number at some college in Alabama. Apparently, he had retired from the Air Force and was now the vice president of a small state university. I waited, tapping a pen nervously on my wooden desk.

"Hello. May I ask who's calling please?"

"I'm an old friend, from California. Is Dr. Marsden available?"

"He's in a meeting at the moment. Shall I interrupt him?"

"No," I answered quickly. "Not at all. I'll call back later."

"Thank you. Oh. I'm sorry, I didn't get your name."

"Oh. Patti Hawn."

Her question caught me off guard. I felt ambushed and immediately sorry to have revealed my name.

"And, if I can please have your number, I'm sure Dr. Marsden would like to speak to you." There was a pause. "He'll be upset if I don't get the number of an old friend."

I gave her my number and quickly hung up. That's not exactly the way I wanted that to go. I would have preferred to be the one in charge. I regretted not being able to take him by surprise. It was funny: after all these years, I was still strategizing moves with this man.

When the phone rang, I knew who it was, but I was still not prepared for the sound of his voice. It was so unquestionably familiar, like I'd just spoken to him yesterday and told him I'd be his date for the prom.

Good Girls Don't

"My God, Patti. Is it really you? Where are you? How are you? How the hell did you find me?"

I forced a little laugh, trying to keep my voice casual and breezy.

"First of all, yes, it is me, and second, I live in California with my husband. Thirdly, I'm pretty damn good on most days and lastly — you weren't so hard to find. I'm a woman on a mission."

"The last time I saw you I think you had joined forces with Jane Fonda and were preparing a march on Washington."

"Yeah, and you were such a hawk I thought you were going to pull out that sword you were wearing and take out your entire graduating class."

That's when he laughed his Santa Claus laugh and the sound filled me up and made my head spin. For some crazy reason I began to hear the Shirelles singing *Will You Still Love Me Tomorrow*, like a stuck record in my brain. I needed time to think.

"Hold the phone a minute," I said. "I have another call."

I put him on hold and took a big swallow of coffee, forcing myself to drink slowly. I walked across the room to the window, concentrating on my breath. I never dreamed he could still have this effect on me.

Robert filled me in on his life. He was on his third marriage, had three daughters and a grandson. He was retired and lived somewhere near Montgomery. I began to tell him my story, describing my life in California, my job as a movie publicist, my husband, my sons. I suddenly felt self-conscious. David was our child and we were still not mentioning it. I remembered the imperceptible weight of his tiny body in my arms, in that fleeting moment before I gave him back to the nurse. I willed myself not to scream.

"Robert, obviously I haven't called you to reminisce. I found our child, our son. His name is David." I picked up speed, urgent to get the words out. "I think I've been working towards this for a long time and want you to know this is completely about me, not you. But I thought I should at least offer you the opportunity to meet him, if you want. No strings."

The silence on his end was so long, I wondered for a second if he'd hung up. I wished I could see his face.

"And there's something else."

"What?" His voice was quiet.

"He's been diagnosed with schizophrenia."

There was a long pause. I guessed I finally got the surprise effect I was hoping for.

"Whew. That's a lot." He faltered. "I don't know — I mean — it's a lot to take in."

"Why don't you talk it over with your wife, your kids, see how everyone feels. I'll be glad to tell you anything, everything or nothing, whatever you decide."

"Wait. Patti. Are you sure you found the right guy?"

I couldn't help but bristle at this question. I was surprised at how proprietary and defensive I was in response to his suggestion.

"There's been no mistake. But I will tell you this. I spent only one day with David in Baltimore, and I felt profoundly moved and changed by the experience..." I trailed off. It was not my job to convince him. "Listen, you don't have to say anything yet, just think about it. If anything I've said strikes a chord, give me a holler."

"Yeah, right. Let me absorb everything. I'll be in touch." He paused. "You know, Patti, I've never for a second forgotten." He paused again, seems unable to finish. "I mean — I always wondered."

I hung up the phone and noticed my hand was trembling.

Nobody was more surprised than I to receive the call several months later offering me a job as the publicist on a movie shooting in Baltimore. The job itself was not a surprise — it's what I did for a living — but the location where it was to be filmed registered as just one more in a long line of coincidences further connecting me to David. The entire production was to be shot just a couple of blocks from where David lived. I'd get to know him differently living so close, I thought. I was packing to leave when Robert's email arrived.

Dearest Patti,

It appears some psychic powers are loose in our worlds. I've felt for a long time that something was happening that touched you and I. I couldn't say this to you on the phone, it would have sounded too crazy, but you've been on my mind again. I say again because these feelings have reoccurred throughout different periods of my life. For some reason, last week, when you called, I actually wasn't that surprised. I felt like I needed to contact you, find you. Something was happening that touched you and I. Of course, I didn't act on my feelings, I rarely do. Thank you for including me in your exciting meeting with David. Believe me, I do not feel pressured! I definitely do not want it to go away! Not again. Your message is full of tragedy and hope and leaves no doubt in my mind of our connection. Your report was tantalizing and I'm anxious to hear more if you have time. What is his last name? Is his mother interested in meeting us? I am intrigued by your description of David. I look forward to learning more and meeting our son soon. Thank you!

Love,
Robert

CHAPTER 27

I WAITED FOR ROBERT IN THE SMALL LIVING ROOM of the old Baltimore apartment I had taken for the duration of the filming, the room lit only by the moon, the yellowish light outlining the odd pieces of worn furniture. I felt lucky to have found this place away from the tourists of the harbor. It could have been someone's home back in the early fifties—the bedroom with twin beds connected by a maple headboard, a low bureau with an attached oval mirror topped with a doily. Even the smell held traces of another era—clean but musty, unused. I carefully placed the family photos, always with me when I'm on location, in strategic spots around the living room. The picture of Steve sat prominently on top of the television and the ones of my kids and the dog on the top of the mahogany bookcase. I went out earlier and shopped for a bottle of good Pinot Noir, but then returned for a bottle of Chablis as well. I had no idea what kind of wine Robert drank, or for that matter if he even drank wine. I'd also bought a large package of Brie and crackers, the European kind that came in a tin, and a bunch of grapes to garnish the cheese. I checked to see if the apartment came equipped with a corkscrew and felt relieved to find one in the drawer.

I wandered into the bathroom, pleased to notice a dimmer on the light switch—a contrast to the rest of the apartment's decidedly dated accoutrements. I turned it down and peered at myself in the mirror before I put my lenses in. My face appeared softer in this light, the signs of age slightly faded. I sighed, slipped in my contacts, decided on pink lipstick and tousled my short curls with my fingertips, trying unsuccessfully to add the texture that Baltimore humidity had stripped from my hair. I continued to stare critically at myself, as women throughout the ages have done before meeting lovers, whether they are past or present. I decided that although my chin was not as firm as it had been, I wore my years well enough.

The doorbell jarred me away from the mirror. He's early, I thought, immediately realizing the irony. I leaned into the door, fixed a smile to my face and opened it wide. I'd forgotten how large he was: a tall man, long thick legs, he filled up the doorway. He wore a stylish navy blue suit, well cut, and a tie with blue and red stripes. He'd grown heavier through his mid-section, a little overweight. He brushed his hair aside in a gesture so familiar; it evoked a memory so strong I felt a physical reaction. His hair, now completely gray, was still thick and wavy, and when he brushed it aside I noticed his hazel eyes, but they looked out of place in this new face. His smell was subtle, like expensive cologne.

In one seamless move he stepped into the room, pulled me into his arms in a big bear hug, and cupped my face with his huge hands. He stared at me so intently it almost knocked me over. And then his big, rumbling, almost-honest laugh filled the room, sounding oddly off key. I squirmed out of his reach, felt awkward as though undressed.

"Look at you," he said. "Time has treated you well."

"It's good to see you, Rob," I said, a bit formally, moving to the center of the room. "You look wonderful. Life seems to have done well by you."

"Life does what life does. I treat myself well. Stand still for a second, girl, let me look at you."

I was surprised that over the next hour, all traces of what he had been, or at least what I thought I remembered, vanished. He might as well have been a complete stranger to me. I tried to recreate a feeling, a longing, anything that would bring him back as my memory wanted him to be. I was surprised how hard I resisted giving up on the faded first love I'd held onto for so long. It had been fueled by some idealistic need, especially since finding David. I wanted to hang on to it just a little longer, but this imposter was making that impossible. I found myself growing irrationally annoyed. Maybe if he were still the Robert of my youth I could present him to David like a beautifully wrapped present: one he could look at and take out to enjoy when he chose. Maybe I could replace the father who died on him.

I poured myself another glass of wine—maybe the third— and studied him, all the while nodding and smiling appropriately. He needed minimal encouragement to talk, his conversation centered mostly on himself. He was in the midst of explaining how tolerant his wife had been throughout their marriage, and even suggested that his youngest daughter reminded him of me at that age. I had begun to wish we could get over this dinner as soon as possible. He had asked practically nothing about David.

I sank into the couch and let the wine spill through me, blotting out his words. I knew I'd had too much to drink. My face felt flushed and unnaturally warm. I got up and walked to the window, and struggled to open it. He was beside me before I even realized he'd gotten up; his arms were around my waist urging me toward him.

"We never had our chance," he said. "Let me stay here with you tonight. I promise you won't regret it."

Waves of rage overtook me with such surprising force that for a moment I lost all sense of control. I jerked away, pushed him so hard he stumbled.

"Get your hands off of me. Why did you come here?" I screamed. "What in the world brought you all these miles? Certainly not to see your son."

My head was spinning out of control as I gulped air from the open window. Robert stood with his hands outstretched as though ready to catch me if I toppled, an expression of shock on his face, which infuriated me even more.

"Patti, I'm so sorry, I just got so caught up in everything. Forgive me, I don't know what happened. I think we've both had too much to drink. Sit down, here, on the couch. I'll get you water. Please calm down. David will be here shortly and I certainly don't want to meet him this way. I came here because I knew it would make you happy. For some reason, when you called, I heard something in your voice, how much you wanted this. I wasn't going to be the guy who disappointed you again. I'm sorry, so sorry."

I made it into the bathroom in time to throw up, continuing to retch long after I had relieved myself of wine and cheese. I sat on the edge of the bathtub staring at its clawed feet, holding a wet towel over my face, hoping for sanity to return. When finally my breathing returned to normal and my head cleared, I realized that David would be here in less than half an hour. For a moment I considered the possibility of not leaving the safety of the clean white bathroom, but I reminded myself that I was not an adolescent; I was a middle-aged woman who has just made a complete fool out of herself. I shuddered to see the ring of mascara that had smeared under my eye, swiped it clean and prepared to face the ridiculous situation that awaited me on the other side of the door.

When I saw Robert standing nervously in the kitchen, washing the wine glasses, I probably saw him truly for the first time since he'd arrived, without the filter of all my baggage. He was a nice, older man who might live down the street. A neighbor, perhaps, who I might nod to at Christmas, but never really try to get to know. He was someone else's husband, belonging to some woman who I'm sure would never be my friend. We would have absolutely nothing in common. I thought of my Steve, with his quick sense of humor and acerbic observations on life. How we could have laughed at this entire scenario, if it had not felt so tragic. Mostly I felt as though I wanted to apologize to this nice man for jumping into the middle of his life.

"Rob, I don't know what came over me. I'm beyond embarrassed."

"No, Patti, please. I'm embarrassed. I was nervous about seeing you and well, I'm a jerk. That's it, plain and simple. I'm sorry, really sorry."

I pictured him getting the phone call from me and realized what a set-up I must have provided. Girl from past enters life of middle-aged man, probably a little bored, with the offer of the possibility to revisit his youth. I never really had the importance in his life that he did in mine, even when we were kids, and certainly not now. How absurd of me to demonize this guy. I couldn't make him wrong for not having paternal feelings toward someone he had rarely thought of after all these years.

"It's me who needs to apologize to you, Robert. This is about me, not you, but mostly it's about David. I think I just needed to find him. You need to know something, though. I'm really flattered that you made a pass at me and who knows — another time, another place — but I'm really in love with my husband. We can't remake the past tonight. Besides, I doubt you and I would have lasted beyond the first year of the Johnson administration."

Robert burst out laughing, only this time it sounded more real. I laughed as well.

For about half an hour, Robert and I acted like parents – even if our son was 40 years old. Robert furtively cleared away all signs of wine and cheese, even put the wine glasses back in the cupboard, as though they might somehow suggest something improper had occurred. Meanwhile, I ran into the bathroom to once again check my face and repair my make up. We behaved like two outdated caricatures of a mom and dad trying to avoid the embarrassment of being caught by their kid in an intimate moment. We felt conspiratorial, even pretended to have something in common, though by now we both knew this was not true.

David arrived right on time, accompanied by one of the counselors from Fellowship House. Funny how being part of a threesome made me more sensitive to David's uniqueness. I was surprised to find myself relieved to see that he was wearing a clean pressed shirt and his shoelaces were tied. Although his misshapen sport coat hung from his thin shoulders as though from a wire hanger, he looked so earnest and somehow pure that once again I was fiercely protective of him. Robert approached David with an outstretched hand, introduced himself, even adding an annoying pat on the back while shaking his hand.

I watched David physically shrink while taking this man in. They exchanged perfunctory greetings, but at no time did I detect anything more than honest curiosity – and even this was clouded by Robert's practiced joviality. David took a seat on the couch next to me. I inched closer to him, like a cat preparing to pounce on every word exchanged between the two of them. When finally I became aware of the absurdity of my behavior and how demeaning this was to David – and for that matter to Robert – I backed off and became a spectator. It occurred to me how little I could find to connect this father and son. David, although above average height, was slender, while Robert was not. While they shared a thick head of hair, neither coloring nor features remotely linked these two physically. Nobody mentioned David's illness or anything pertaining to his past. It was as if Robert was meeting a prospective college applicant for the first time; he was appropriate but dry, unemotional.

"I heard you like philosophy," David said, once again surprising me, taking the initiative in the conversation.

"Yeah, well sort of, I guess. That was such a long time ago, back in college. I can barely remember. I've made my career in the Air Force, as I'm sure your mother, I mean, Patti, has told you. I'm retired now and head up a college in Alabama. I used to get back to these parts more often, but now, I have no reason. Family's gone." He gave a short uncomfortable laugh. "Last year I became an official at the college."

Had he always been so stuffy? I can't tell if it's his age or just the way he's put together. I'd forgotten how he spoke when he was a kid.

David, who started off so brilliantly, was beginning to shut down. He did not possess the guile to camouflage his feelings, and gave a loud yawn. Robert shot me an odd look as though to ask what to say next.

"I'm starved, guys," I said with determined cheer. "Let's move on to the restaurant. I can't wait to taste good old Maryland seafood."

We drove to the restaurant, Robert and I in the front seat, our son in the back, pretending we were a normal family. There were no prodding questions or proclamations of amazement at the strangeness of any of it. And that, of course, made it even stranger.

I wish I could say the evening got better—that there were epiphanies, or at least connections. When David refused to be drawn into any conversation and withdrew completely, Robert gave up all pretense of interest and spoke only to me. I failed miserably at attempts to draw David out and finally drifted into my own thoughts while poor Robert droned on about his golf game.

I found peculiar memories popping out during this supremely awkward meal. For a second I entertained the thought of retracing my steps back to that huge left turn I took when I became pregnant. I pictured myself wearing Robert's class ring scotch-taped around my finger, dancing in my green tulle gown with the dyed-to-match shoes. I remembered how everything then was dyed-to-match, so predictable. I recalled my girlhood bedroom with Robert's initials carved into my maple headboard and how angry Mom was when she discovered it.

Back in the apartment, after Robert had left, David and I sat on the couch. Now that it was just the two of us, the slightly catatonic look had left his face.

"Are you disappointed?" I asked. "Is he what you imagined?"

David shrugged. "I've always felt the womb was more important than the sperm."

The swiftness with which he delivered this line took me completely by surprise. Sometimes our past collides into the present with such heartbreaking clarity it makes your heartbeat stutter.

"David," I said, and my tentativeness got his immediate attention. "I've been thinking about that question you asked when we were walking. You asked why I decided on adoption with you. No. It's OK. I want to talk about it. I don't know the answer, but I'm trying to understand."

Damn. I thought I had worked this out in my head better than this. I didn't want to be confused on this issue; at least I didn't want to appear confused to David.

"I was told to forget you. Everyone told me to. Part of me said 'screw them,' but part of me believed them. Believed that they knew best. And so, I sort of buried you away in a box—but I guess you sort of kept pecking at me, like a chick in a shell."

I shook my head, exhausted. My eyes were closed and my

fingers were rubbing my forehead. It was all I could say. I was surprised to hear a soft, rich laugh coming from David. I looked up into his smiling blue eyes.

"Like in a chick in shell," he said. "I like that."

We sat there on the couch for a while in silence. Then David spoke.

"So. When did I start pecking?"

"I don't know," I said, shaking my head. I was too tired for this. Then, everything rushed back to me. Random images began making static appearances inside my head. Mountains came into my mind, a Chinese restaurant with mom across the table from me, the way Malibu looked from my window the day I married Steve. "The pecking started long ago," I told David.

CHAPTER 28

I sink deep into the large cushy train seat and let the clicking of the wheels lull me somewhere in the midst of yesterday and today. Like that of an ancient Tibetan bowl, the sound releases trapped memories. It's easy to forget where the train comes from or where it delivers me because I float suspended inside a sacred spot called in-between. Blurred telephone poles, faded factories, all ask if they are real. But inside this mighty capsule of steel and smoke where options are few, I rest. Here, there is nothing to control. I am free to tiptoe gently back through time, not rush and calculate as is my usual way.

IT WAS LATE FEBRUARY; I'd been freezing on a movie set in New York for a week when I received the phone call from David's caretaker, Bob, in Baltimore. I'd had many conversations with him over the past several years and was happy to be included in David's life, although I struggled with such a strange role, never exactly sure where or when to step in. David's mother was still unwilling to meet me, although apparently she didn't disapprove of David's and my relationship. In many ways it was a time of terrible frustration. I like to think that I'm a capable, intelligent woman who makes things happen, but in David's case I felt as though I was operating with both hands and feet bound tightly together. I had to constantly remind myself that David had a mother who was obviously in charge of his welfare; I walked a fine line, to hold myself back. Bob seemed to understand my dilemma and most of the time he included me in what was going on. But the call from him on this Friday afternoon was the first time I'd really heard how David's illness could manifest itself, and it filled me with trepidation.

Bob's voice on the other end of my cell had been terse, straight to the point. If I have to have bad news, I've always believed that's the best way to get it.

"David's been hospitalized. A psychotic episode. They kept him for about a week, but he's better now. He was released this morning. They changed his medication, so they're watching him until they can see what's up. Seems to be doing O.K. but I thought you'd want to know."

After the call, I was filled with a dreadful sense of catastrophe looming. It was easy to believe that nothing was wrong with David. After all, I hadn't been there during the really rough years. Up until now I'd been spared anything other than the sometimes-odd physical effects caused by his medication. Bob had said that his medication had been changed, so maybe that was all it took, but I knew little about his disease and had never fully trusted the diagnosis since nobody could ever find a history of schizophrenia in either Robert's or my families. I had suspected that his illness had been triggered by early drug use, but information was sketchy. I only knew what David himself had told me, and who knows how reliable that was.

I'd called David at the halfway house and told him I would be arriving at the train station in Baltimore at 5 p.m. He quickly agreed to meet me. I decided to suspend any questions until I could see him and evaluate his condition for myself.

As soon as I finished my work for the day, I threw a few

things in a suitcase and grabbed a cab to Penn Station. I was so pre-occupied by thoughts of David's illness that a man on a bike almost hit me when I got out of the cab. I hurried into the station and found my way to the track just in time to see the train burrowing toward me. I followed a group of Friday-night commuters and grabbed a seat by the window, where I settled in for the three-hour ride to Baltimore.

I immediately plunged into darkness as the train bore through a tunnel leading us out of the city. As I leaned back into the seat, I allowed the comfort of the train sounds to soothe me, waited for my mind to soften and the memories to find me. I couldn't help but remember another train ride, a lifetime ago, when I was a young frightened girl carrying a baby inside me. I barely recognized her. Yet, here I was today going to see that baby. My hand instinctively reaches inside my loosened parka and I touch my belly — almost as though I could bring back that girl. I couldn't help but wonder who she might have become without that unwanted pregnancy.

A rainstorm broke over the string of abandoned factories that dotted the New Jersey Landscape; the sudden downpour splashed heavy sheets of water over the old brick buildings. Gusts of wind lashed the bare trees, bending them toward the ground.

The events that were set in motion the day I handed the infant David back to the hospital nurse forty years ago determined a path for me. I always felt that I'd claimed my life as my own the day I left Maryland and moved to California. But maybe it was really the moment I defied everyone and visited the forbidden maternity ward to see my baby.

The train glided into a town somewhere outside of Trenton and a pair of well-dressed young men boarded, chatting loudly about a reception they would attend later that night in Washington. Their voices, loud, intrusive, forced me to stare out the window, where the winter haze had thickened over the color-less city into a pre-dusk murkiness. The landscape, although achingly beautiful, today felt bleak, enveloped me in sadness. I had such an ambivalent relationship with the East Coast. I secret-ly believed that only grown-ups were allowed to live here. It was as though my life was sliced right down the middle—the first half lived as an adult and the second half as a kid.

Soon the rain turned to drizzle; the lightning was sporadic, distant. The railroad tracks ran along a river that curved out of sight, behind the tall trees. The river appeared again, flowed in gentle curves past a small town somewhere outside of Philadelphia. A flat, sandy inlet surrounded by gloomy old weep-ing willows blurred the landscape into a dream.

I wondered if I would have gotten pregnant so soon with Michael if I hadn't been trying to replace what had been taken from me. Or, if I would have fought so hard to marry Eric Donovan, without that first pregnancy. Sometimes life seemed determined by cosmic blueprint stamped out by family history, but the truth was that every time I took control and followed my instincts, it changed my path. Mom's mother and her child had died during childbirth; my own mother lost her first-born and apparently felt forced into a marriage to Daddy. I could have easi-ly lived out a destiny prescribed by them, but I didn't. I'm con-vinced that the day that I decided to search for David changed that blueprint.

The coincidences, if that's what they were, that connected me to David still astound me. What strange force led me to become a drug counselor at the same place where David might have gone for help when he was a kid, or led me to climb the Masada in Israel while he lived there in a kibbutz? I pulled my coat more tightly around me when I thought about his time as an Orthodox Jew, when he sat with the corpses at the Takoma Park Funeral Home to usher them out of this world into the next — the same funeral home that held Mom's body only a few years later. What led me to that bookstore that took me to Nepal and began the dreams that awakened my desire to find him?

Somehow I found comfort in these memories; I was reminded that there is something much more powerful at work than anything I can make happen. In the end we all have our own paths. I can't change the past or fix David, but what I can do is love him and be a part of his life.

It was nearly five p.m. when the train pulled through the veiled fog into Baltimore and screeched to a halt. A gust of moist air sent a chill over my shoulder as I hurried onto the platform and into the small station. The terminal was deserted, so it was easy to spot David seated by himself at the end of the empty bench. I saw him before he saw me. He was so pale he looked blue. He was smoking fast, inhaling every couple of seconds. There were bags under his eyes. His head kept jerking slightly — the medication, probably. If I expected him to be ranting about aliens or making public speeches about Jesus or any extreme stereotypes I might have harbored, I was mistaken. He just looked small. I'd grown used to seeing David looking disheveled, wearing dirty clothes, even needing deodorant, but I wasn't prepared for how thin he looked. His face had become gaunt and his wrists hung out from under the sleeves of his filthy army jacket like sticks. There was a relief, though, in finally seeing him — even in this state.

By the time I reached him he was standing, smiling thinly at me. Wordlessly I walked into his outstretched arms and laid my head on his shoulder. It was as though I was holding a bird with a broken wing. When he craned his neck as far away from me as it would go, I could feel rather than see that I needed to give him time to trust me again. This took me by surprise; from the beginning we'd always been so easy together, even effortless.

"It's good to see you," I said, looking directly into his eyes, trying not to betray any fear I might have. "You've been through an ordeal. I'm glad it's over."

I guess it was the right thing to say: an audible sigh of relief escaped from him David the beginning of his beautiful smile spread to his eyes.

"I wish Bob hadn't called you," he said. "It's kinda embarrassing."

"Hardly anything to be embarrassed about, David. It happened, it's over, and we don't need to talk about it if you don't want to. Just know I'm available if you want me to be. You should know I asked Bob to let me know stuff about you. I'm not just a fair-weather mom, you know."

I let the silence between us settle in for a while as we climbed into a cab. I told the driver to take us to the harbor and watched David edge himself as far as he could into the corner of the car.

"How are you feeling?" I asked. "Do the new meds agree with you?"

"Yeah, they're all right," he shrugged. "They gave me a roommate and I, well, that's when it started to happen…" His voice trailed off. I saw him stiffen as he searched for words to complete his sentence. Then he snickered, and mumbled something I didn't catch.

"What'd you say?" But he didn't answer.

Neither of us said anything else for maybe two or three minutes. I finally broke the silence.

"Lousy weather," I said.

"Do you believe in God?" he asked, ignoring my weather statement as though I had never spoken.

"Sometimes," I answered. "Why?"

"I dunno, just wondered. She wants me to get a vasectomy. "

"Who?" I asked.

"My mother. She's been, ummm …" he finished unintelligibly.

He was talking loudly. "I get mad sometimes when she says that. Brings it up a lot."

I had refrained from anything other than perfunctory questions regarding his mother during the time we had known one another, but when he said this, I wanted to scream out that she was wrong. You can't take away someone's dignity like that. I didn't answer him at first. I fumbled around for some response that wouldn't trigger huge emotions. I was trying to formulate an answer when I looked over at David's lined, joyless face. He was staring out the window of the car, pulling away again. He began another statement, something about an accident he'd seen down at the harbor. Only he couldn't find the word for harbor. It was as though his sentences would unravel somewhere in the middle. His mind was running all over the place, and I was scared to death about what he would say next. Then I said something I hadn't planned on. "Yes, David, I do believe in God, at least most of the time. Today I do."

I kept my eyes straight ahead as we got out of the cab and together into the chilled evening. I asked him if he wanted to walk a bit and he nodded. My emotions were all over the place, and the welcome cold helped clear my mind. We trudged up the steps onto St. Paul Street and began the long walk toward the touristy harbor. David was out of shape, winded from his hospital stay or medication. The air slapped across our faces, and it wasn't long before he broke the silence again by asking me if I would lend him money. He had never asked this before. I asked him how much he needed and he said five dollars.

By the time I reached into my purse, he'd forgotten and moved on to something else, beginning sentences, and then struggling like someone who severely stutters, desperately searching for the end of his thought. I began to wonder if going into a public restaurant was the right move, but decided to try it. We needed to eat.

We moved into a crowded seafood restaurant, one that we'd been to before, decorated with a large brightly lit aquarium. All the lights and jostling crowds made him shrink a little. He kept jerking his head as though he was trying to shake something away. By the time the waitress took our order, David was talking in an unnaturally loud voice. "I want a hamburger, with onions," he got out. The busy waitress stared down at David, seeing him for the first time.

"Sure, sweetie, you can have anything you'd like," her voice condescending, she gave me a knowing look.

I wanted to tell him to lower his voice. It had been a mistake to come here. I didn't know David this way. I felt scared. Felt like running away. What if this accelerated into something I couldn't handle? I made a mental note to remember where Bob's phone number was in case things got out of hand. When I looked into David's face and saw the dark raccoon-like circles under his eye, as hard as I tried to meet his gaze, my eyes bounced away.

The sigh he let out found its way into my gut. "Do you have a cigarette?" he mumbled.

"You know I don't smoke, David. I'll get the waitress to buy us a pack if you want one."

He cut me off mid-sentence. "Why did you come here?"

"To see you. Now that you're in my life, well, I guess it's a done deal. Unless you tell me not to come, I'll be here. Do you want me to stop coming?"

David closed his eyes. His lips moved and his voice became quiet. "No, that's not what I want. I guess I'm still fighting the meds I have to take. After all these year, I've never gotten used to taking them."

And just like that he was back. Finally, he had said something I knew how to answer. "The meds are a lifeline for you," I said. "I'm sure the side-effects are tough but the alternatives are worse. It'll probably be a day or two for you to start feeling better; but I'd like to hang out with you today, and together we'll just take it as it comes. What do you say?"

"Tell the waitress to get me some cigarettes and a cup of coffee," he responded. His hand moved to cover up a huge yawn that escaped from his body like trapped air, and after that he seemed to settle into a less agitated state.

"I know I have to take them," he continued. "Don't know why I fight it. They make me think better and I sure need all the help I can get to find a job."

I sat there unable to think of anything else to say. I bent down to tie my shoelace so he wouldn't see the tears that filled my eyes. I saw, for a moment, a flicker of his pain, which until now had remained hidden from me. It was also clear to me that I could not fix him. And that was the hardest of all — because God knows I am my mother's daughter, a fixer.

We spent the rest of the afternoon walking in the light rain around the harbor. We stopped in a bookstore, where he drank more coffee and smoked more cigarettes, and then sat on a bench under my umbrella, watching the boats. I pointed out a jogger who was running around the harbor and a sailboat out at sea, but for the most part we said nothing. Although we were both drenched he seemed content to sit there. His breath sounded more regular, and although he yawned frequently, I could sense he was growing quieter inside.

There was something peaceful about the two of us just sitting quietly together in the afternoon rain. I finally stopped talking and let the mist fall around us like a cloud. I had given up something that apparently needed to be set free that afternoon: my expectations. I had harbored some arrogant notion that I could love away

David's illness, that I could take away his pain; make him into something else other than who he was. I realized that afternoon that I had set my own agenda apart from him. He was perfect exactly the way he was. All I could do was be with him, honor and love him.

By the time I returned to California, David was taking his medication regularly again, and the next time we spoke he was taking a bus an hour away each way to work as a dishwasher at a local restaurant. He told me he enjoyed the ride each morning. It gave him time to think about things, and he was making his own money. We never spoke again about the vasectomy. That was between him and his mother, and although I strongly disagreed with her, I successfully fought the urge to become involved. It proved to be a good decision because apparently the problem went away without any intrusion from me.

Good Girls Don't

CHAPTER 29

IN OCTOBER THE HEAT GIVES WAY to the best weather that southern California has to offer. Summer is over, but I still need to be reminded when one season becomes another. You have to pay attention. Like today, the sky and the ocean were both so blue they looked neon. Roses were still in bloom but they didn't smell the same as they did last month. They didn't smell at all. The best part about October at the beach is the air. It was clear and clean, and smelled a little like Mom's sheets on the clothesline when I was a kid back in Maryland.

As I drove along the coast to the airport, I watched the tiny surfers who dotted the ocean. With sadness, I turned away from the ocean into the formidable network of Los Angeles International Airport. I eased my Camry into a space in one of the vast parking structures and glanced at my watch. I had to chuckle at myself. In the past, I'd always waited until the last minute to get to airports. But not today. David was coming to visit me and I wanted to make sure to be the first face he saw when he got off the plane.

I hurried through the crowded terminal and scanned the arrival board. Flashing lights alerted me that his flight had been transferred to another terminal. I made a quick decision to walk the quarter mile or so to the other side of the airport, but then realized it would probably make me late. After some anxious calculations I realized it would definitely make me late. His plane was probably landing right now. I plunged back into the street, clanging against a public trashcan, almost knocking it over. I had a disturbing vision of David wandering around the airport, maybe wondering if I'd forgotten him.

Maybe he'd think that anyone who could forget him when he was a baby could do the same thing again at the airport. It took very little time for my mind to start unhinging. Fifteen minutes later, I'd convinced myself that either David was hopelessly lost, frightened, wandering the airport looking for me, or he'd entered into a full-blown psychotic episode and the police had picked him up. All my fault. I should never have sent for him. What a colossal mistake I'd made. By this time I'd reached the baggage claim where I thought we had agreed to meet.

There were long lines everywhere, but I spotted an old guy with a badge pinned to his shirt. I explained to him that I was here to meet someone who might have a disability and he may be lost. I immediately felt I had betrayed David by saying this. Actually David had made his way all over the world, probably was a savvier traveler than I was—and besides, anyone who'd navigated the streets for much of his life could surely find his way around an airport. The old guy wasn't much help and I moved on, panning feverishly across the landscape of moving people.

Why didn't I allow for more time? I asked myself. I was a complete fool to think this would go smoothly.

My throat was so dry it felt glued together. I began searching for the police to report David missing while calling Maryland on my cell phone to speak to anyone at the halfway house, although I had no idea what I'd say when, or if, I even reached anyone.

It had taken me exactly 20 minutes to enter into a full-out panic attack. And then I spotted him. He was standing right under the American Airlines sign, exactly where he should be, smiling easily, although the smile rapidly faded into concern when he saw me. He put his thin arm around my shoulder and drew me to him.

"Calm down," he said. "I'm fine. It's the plane that couldn't find the right terminal, not me. I just called and left a message on your machine where to find me." He kissed me on the forehead, on the place where my hair parts, and led me out into the street.

As we walked into the parking lot I couldn't help but think what an odd-looking couple we were. I was dressed in designer jeans, a short leather jacket. David was wearing stained work pants a couple of sizes too big for him, a long-sleeved cotton shirt with two missing buttons, dirty sneakers with one gray sock and one grayer sock. His hair was badly in need of cutting, and his glasses sat lopsided on his face, held together with scotch tape. He'd lost weight since I'd last seen him and needed a dentist. He had a definite hygiene problem that had clearly held him back with jobs. We'd talked about this in the past and his response was always the same: "Yeah, yeah, I know. I have to work on that."

"I haven't planned anything special," I said. "Thought we'd let the weekend unfold. See where it takes us."

David nodded in agreement.

"I like that," he said, as I knew he would.

"Although, I know for sure one place it's going to take us," I continued. "To the barber shop."

David was not remotely offended by my bluntness. I think he'd grown to expect it. Even like it.

It always amazed me how easily we fell into a rhythm together. In the past several years we'd seen each other dozens of times. I initiated subjects of conversation, often in the form of questions, and David provided the answers, usually sparse and often surprising. We were both very comfortable with this arrangement.

"You look thin. Are you eating?" I asked, aware that my remark was a stereotypical mother question, but unable to help myself. I began to plan pasta dishes with extra cheese and maybe split pea soup with fresh carrots.

"I just make easy stuff," he said. "I guess I haven't felt much like cooking anything lately. I've been working helping out on construction sites and have to get up so early in the morning to get jobs that by the time I get home I'm too tired to cook." It was times like this that I had an overwhelming desire to swoop him up and bring him to California. I'd move him into my house and do nothing but cook for him. I'd make sure his socks matched and his clothes were clean and he would never have to wear glasses that were scotch-taped together. Fat and warm, that's how I'd keep him.

I remembered a previous visit, when I had asked David to tell me about when he first knew he was sick. His answer haunted me still.

"I was living on the streets of Chicago," he stated simply. "I was homeless. It was cold. The cold made me crazy."

And it had nearly driven me crazy to hear those words. To imagine your child cold and hungry, at any age, is agonizing to a mother.

My daydream of nourishing this thin man fizzled and reality took its place. I knew that David had a mother already, and I'd learned to respect that. I'd known from the beginning that this was not my right. My job was not to fix or change anything. All I could do was be David's friend, but I must admit to sometimes moving awkwardly between friend and mother. I knew this was a kind of purgatory that would always be a part of this journey.

We pulled into my garage and I noticed Steve's bike hanging on the wall, exactly where it had been for two years. I'm not sure why I noticed it today, but I did.

"When's the last time you were on a bike?" I blurted out. "You can use that one and we can explore the beach. What do you think?"

David looked at me like I'd just asked him to climb aboard my helicopter for a short spin.

"It's been a long time since I've been on a bike," he responded. "I think the last time, I was about 13."

"C'mon. If I can ride a bike, so can you," I pushed. "Nothing to it. Comes back to you just like sex." He did a double take and then broke into a laugh. He obviously didn't expect this from me. His deep, true laugh had the power to shift moods and clear the air.

"OK," he said finally. "Let me practice first and we'll go."

Manhattan Beach was a perfect little beach town. My kids called it Pleasantville. It sometimes made you wonder if central casting was involved in placing all the beautiful blonde people into strategic spots along the tree-lined residential roads and, of course, along the wide, sandy beach. My husband often joked that we would probably be too old to be allowed onto the beach in a couple of years. When I moved here some twenty years ago I was a single mom and thought I'd died and gone to heaven. It was a sleepy little surf community then, known for its abundance of airline pilots and flight attendants who were infamous for their ability to party. During the 80's it was a town of sex, drugs and rock and roll, and by the nineties it had been discovered by young families with children who liked the schools. I'd lived here through it all, and on most found it about as nice a life as I could dream of.

I tried to imagine David's first impression of this place as we rode our bikes through the quaint streets and manicured front yards. He'd just left Baltimore, a town certainly not without its own kind of charm, but clearly opposite of this. I was impressed that David was handling the bike with such confidence. I liked seeing him ride through the streets, often taking the lead, a new experience for him.

When we stopped at Starbucks for a coffee I noticed something different about him. The muscles in his face, around his eyes and even his jaw had relaxed. The medicine he took made his face appear tense, but today he looked peaceful. The ocean breeze lifted his long hair off of his face, and for the first time I noticed a strong jaw etched into his profile. The corner of his mouth, which he habitually stretched into contortions — also an effect of the medication — fell into a softer, more natural pose. It was as though, for a moment, a veil had lifted and I could see into who he might have been.

We didn't speak, but he looked at me longer than usual, and I saw the smile behind his eyes. We sat outside of Starbucks, our legs dangling from the wall, and watched the beautiful people pass us by.

"Is it a requirement to be blonde to live here?" he asked.

"Yes, but you're related to me so it's OK."

We sat at Starbucks for over an hour, discussing all kinds of stuff. We talked about the different kinds of seashells in California and debated the best place to get crab cakes in Maryland. We described to one another all the different colors of mornings we'd noticed in all the many places we'd both visited.

"Once I climbed the Masada in Israel at dawn," I said. "I'll never forget the morning light. I actually became a kind of born-again-Jew for a minute."

"I spent a whole year in a kibbutz in Israel," David offered, as a matter of fact. "I didn't climb the Masada but I worked in an orange grove near Jerusalem and had to get up at dawn every morning to pick the oranges. The morning light made the oranges look red." He paused. "I once went to the adoption agency — to find you. Well, not exactly to find you, more to find out if you were

Jewish. I was heavy into Hassidic Judaism at the time. I was working at the Takoma Park Funeral Home. I was the guy who sat with the dead people for the first twenty-four hours after they died. It's a really holy job and I wasn't even sure I was really a Jew."

I was no longer surprised at the odds and ends of David's life. Of course a million questions crowded into my brain at once. Was he sick during this time? What stirred him toward such a fundamental look at religion? What took him to Israel? How long did he stay? Was he alone? My God, I remembered what he'd told me about his work at the same funeral home that prepared my mother's body for burial just eight years ago. But I said nothing. Today, I didn't ask. I knew that David let me into his world on his time, when he was ready. I'd learned a little about patience from him — not an easy lesson for me.

Our conversation floated effortlessly. For a while we were not different, not mother and son, man and woman, not even friends, just two souls connected by warm sun and soft air. For a moment, I thought of this man who sat beside me today, on his 41st birthday, and remembered the infant I'd held in my arms, who I promised to never forget.

"What would you do if someone gave you a million dollars?" I asked.

I had no idea where this question came from. I'd never heard David ask for anything. He had never mentioned a television set or a stereo or an article of clothing that he longed for. He owned so little, his few meager belongings usually left somewhere along his way. Once I bought him a CD player and a gift certificate to a music store but he never redeemed it, just never got around to it. Another time I bought him a thick fleece jacket with Tommy Hilfiger's name sewn into the front of it. I never saw him wear the jacket and I suspected it was probably left somewhere in one of the many places David had lived since I'd known him.

"I never get to buy you anything," I said. There must be something that turns you on. Something you absolutely can't live without."

"Nah, I'm fine," he answered. "I can't think of anything I want. Maybe a cup of coffee."

David's addiction to caffeine was daunting. I'd seen him go through several huge cups at one sitting. I thought it might have something to do with the side effects of his medicine. He didn't know it, but I'd bought him a $50.00 gift certificate to Starbucks, which I planned to give to him later that night.

I threw my hands up in mock despair and told him I'd have no trouble filling up a wish list if given a million dollars. David just smiled in that secret way that made me feel he knew something I didn't. I was starting to think he did.

We made our way down to the bike path, along the ocean, to begin our journey. The day was extraordinary. It was a palette of salt-water taffy. Whitecaps spit phosphorescent particles into streaks of pink and silver waves. One moment the water was the color of lavender and the next that of a field of sage. We guided our bikes directly into the warm sunlight and lifted our chins to catch the ocean breeze. David passed me without noticing. We saw a group of suntanned teenage boys stop their volleyball game to watch a stunning, bikini-clad redhead stroll the beach with the entitlement of ownership that only the young and beautiful possess. A young mother jogged on the path pushing twin babies in a carriage, and a father, with his son, dug into a sand dune with paper cups, building a castle. A group of middle-aged women walked on the soft sand lifting their legs as though in a parade. I caught up to David and rode along beside him for a second or two. We both turned at the same time to hear a salsa band playing inside of one of the houses that lined the strand. A breeze gently pushed against our backs, making the trip even more effortless.

We soared as though our wheels never touched the ground, grazing the sides of the sand, weaving gracefully as though we were dancing a tango. I couldn't remember another time in my life when time had hung quite so endlessly.

I pulled up beside David and got a full view of his face as he pedaled, making a wide turn against the edge of the path. He'd picked up a little speed and was handling the bike as though it was an extension of his body. He looked all polished and shiny from the sun, as joyous as any human being I'd ever seen. I stared at him so hard I almost crashed into him, but he slightly turned the handlebars, expertly navigating his bike to avoid me. He threw back his head and laughed with the pure joy of the moment.

"Remember what you asked me a while back?" he yelled over his shoulder.

"I asked you lots of things," I shouted back.

"That thing about the million dollars," he said. "You know, like what would I buy?"

"Oh yeah. Did you decide?"

"Yeah," he said, turning serious. "A bike."

Minutes later, we were in Hermosa Beach; we paused near the pier to catch our breath and people-watch. I pointed eastward, up the block.

"There's the bookstore I told you about," I said, pointing at the *Either/Or* sign, barely within sight. "That's where the book on Nepal found me."

David nodded and then his eyes glazed a bit, and I knew his mind had caught an edge. I waited a few minutes and then, despite my efforts, I nudged him.

"What are you thinking?"

"You didn't try to find me after Nepal," he said. "I guess I'm still wondering why you finally did it."

I couldn't give him an answer. Before meeting him, I might

have tried to make something up, invented an explanation, and babbled until I tired us both out. Today, though, I just smiled at him and shook my head slightly. "It just seemed the right time."

And my son smiled back.

good girls Don't

Made in the USA
Lexington, KY
03 December 2011